Visual Diagnosis

SELF-TESTS ON RHEUMATOLOGY

The Continuing Medical Education Series on Visual Diagnosis Self-tests.

MERIT PUBLISHING INTERNATIONAL

European address:

35 Winchester Street
Basingstoke
Hampshire
RG21 7EE
U.K.
TEL: (1256) 841008
FAX: (1256) 841099

North American address:

8260 N.W. 49th Manor
Pine Grove
Coral Springs
Florida 33067
U.S.A.
TEL: (954) 755-4280
FAX: (954) 755-4287

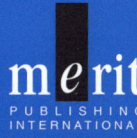

merit
PUBLISHING
INTERNATIONAL

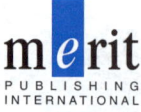

merit
PUBLISHING
INTERNATIONAL

Visual Diagnosis

SELF-TESTS RHEUMATOLOGY

PAUL EMERY

CHRISTINA JOHNSON

CHARLES RICHARDSON

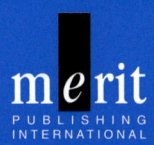

merit
PUBLISHING
INTERNATIONAL

CONTENTS

VISUAL DIAGNOSIS : RHEUMATOLOGY

Rheumatology is concerned with the study of diseases which affect the locomotor system. These include: arthritis, soft tissue bone disease and conditions of soft tissue and bone. All of these may be a consequence of degenerative or inflammatory disease.

Most of these conditions are seen worldwide. Degenerative and inflammatory disease are common in both community and hospital medicine.

It is important to realise that symptomatic joint disease may relate to disease in other body systems and this represents the single most important factor in determining disability in later life. A feature common to all (or the vast majority) of these conditions is pain. This may arise from the joints, periarticular tissues and bone. A simple classification of the conditions studied in rheumatology is shown.

In general terms, the aim of treatment in rheumatology is to reduce the pain and suffering of joint disease. This is achieved by both symptomatic treatment and, increasingly, with the use of therapies which influence and suppress the disease processes themselves. The ultimate aim of therapy is to prevent disability in later life. Indeed, it has been argued that rheumatoid arthritis is the commonest cause of potentially treatable disability in the Western world. Therefore it becomes important to diagnose accurately and treat this condition.

Classification of conditions causing joint pain
Osteoarthritis
Septic arthritis
Crystal deposition disease
Reactive arthritis
Rheumatoid arthritis
Ankylosing spondylitis
Vasculitis*
Dermatomyositis*
SLE*
Scleroderma characterised by joint pain alone
*In these conditions joint pain is a part of a wider clinical picture.

Bone disease (commonly presenting to rheumatologists)
Paget's Disease
Osteoporosis
Osteomalacia.

Soft tissue rheumatism
Simple mechanical back pain
Fibromyalgia
Rotator cuff disease of the shoulder
Polymyalgiarheumatica.

In recent years there have been a number of key developments which have greatly improved the ability of rheumatologists to treat many of these conditions effectively. These developments can be divided into improved techniques to diagnose, predict outcome (and hence tailor therapy) and the availability of more effective therapy. Of course these developments are dependent on an increased knowledge of the basic pathological processes underlying rheumatic disease.

Individual advances worthy of a special mention include:

- Magnetic resonance imaging to provide high quality images of joint and bone anatomy
- Musculoskeletal ultrasound to provide bedside images of joint and periarticular tissues
- Increased use of arthroscopy to visualise joint pathology directly
- The use of genetic markers to identify patients with a poor prognosis in RA
- Accurate markers for monitoring the progress of patients with autoimmune disease
- Increased understanding of the immunology of inflammatory processes
- The development of rational therapies for the treatment of autoimmune disease
- The development of specific chondroprotective agents which may be able to influence the natural outcome of OA.

Despite these advances, and the help that they provide clinicians, it should be remembered that the diagnosis and treatment of articular and peri articular conditions remains dependent on good clinical skills combined with knowledge of regional anatomy and pathological processes. Clearly, these clinical skills are required by both hospital specialists and the primary care physicians who refer patients to them.

In this book we provide a series of case histories, illustrated with photographs and investigations, to cover the most important and common rheumatological conditions. Each case history is followed by a series of questions, with the answers on the following page. This cannot be a substitute for bedside learning but certainly can provide a useful adjunct.

CASE 1

A 60-year-old man attends your clinic complaining of pain in his hands. 'I've had arthritis for years', he says. An X-ray of his hands is arranged.

Describe the features shown on the X-ray.

What is the diagnosis?

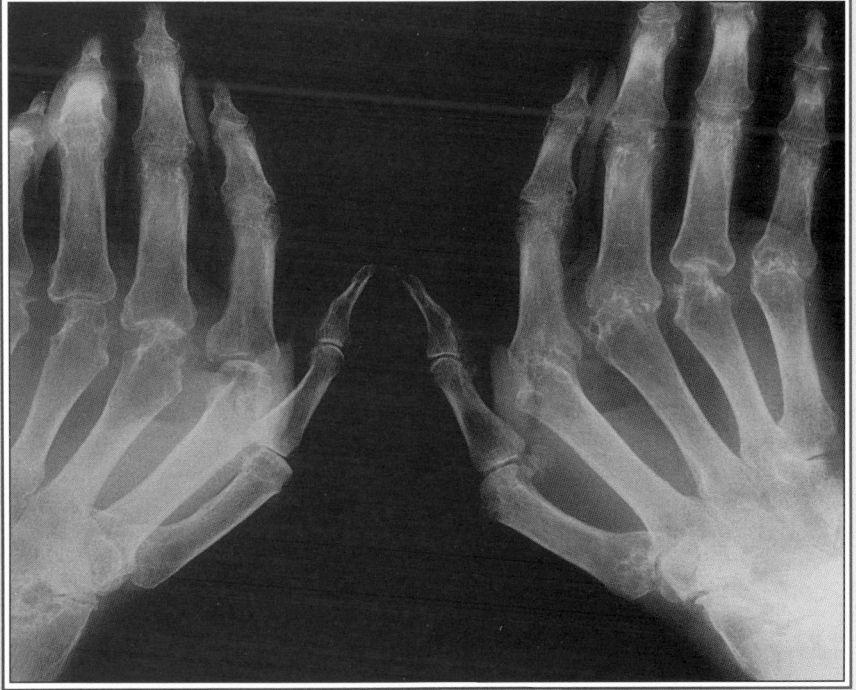

X-ray of hands

Answer to Case 1

The radiological hallmarks of established rheumatoid arthritis are:

- Symmetrical involvement of the small joints - MCP, PIP, and MTP joints

- Soft tissue swelling

- Periarticular osteoporosis

- Loss of joint space

- Bony erosions. (See Figure 1).

Ultimately the combination of progressive joint disease associated with inflammation of the surrounding tendons and ligaments may result in joint instability and the development of deformities. The joint deformities most commonly seen are:

- Subluxation (partial dislocation) at the wrist and MCP joints

- Ulnar deviation of the fingers

- Swan neck deformity

- Boutonniere deformity. (See Figure 2).

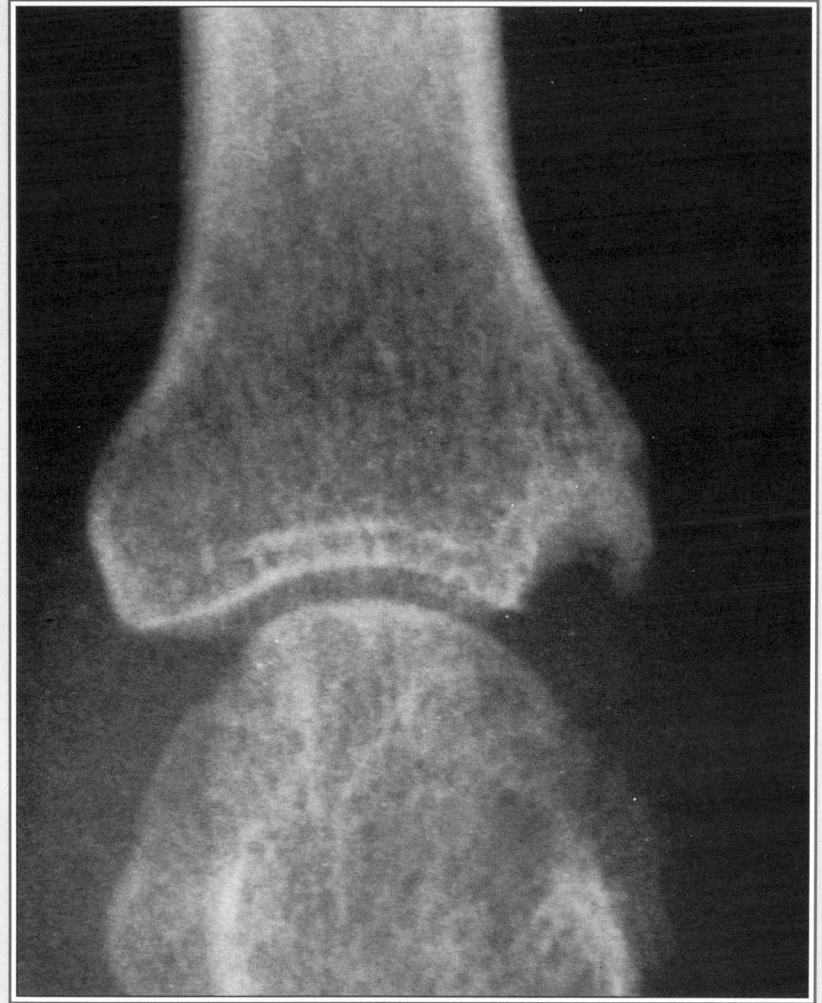

Figure 1: Close up of a joint erosion

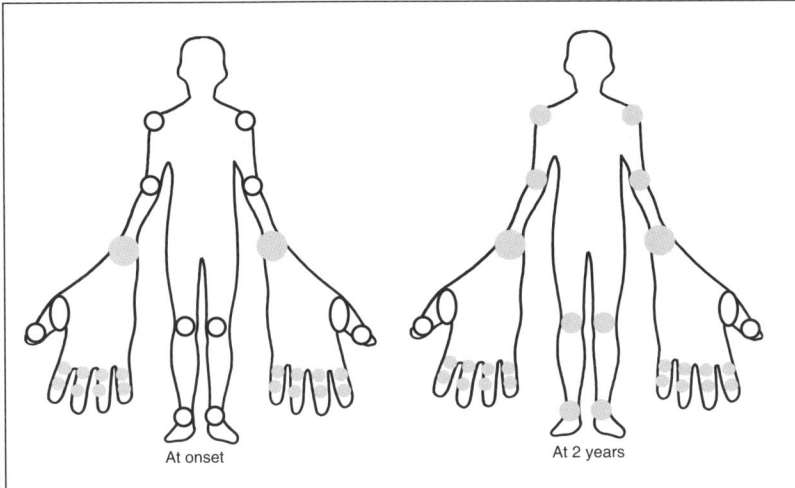

At onset

At 2 years

Figure 2: Progressive joint involvement in rheumatoid arthritis

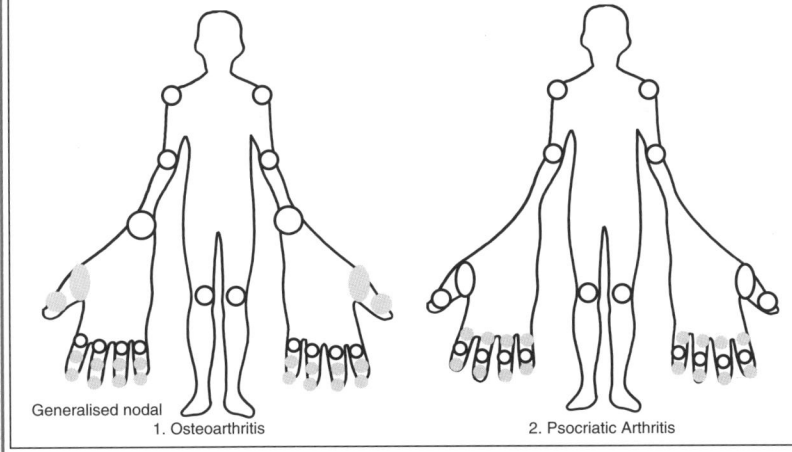

Generalised nodal
1. Osteoarthritis

2. Psocriatic Arthritis

Figure 3: Hand joint involvement in rheumatic diseases

The homonuculus illustrates the pattern of joint progression involvement in rheumatoid arthritis, and contrasts hand joint involvement in 3 diseases. (See Figures 2 & 3).

There are a number of aspects to the treatment to be considered in a patient with established RA:

Symptomatic

The non steroidal anti-inflammatory drugs (NSAIDs) provide the cornerstone of symptomatic treatment. They inhibit the production of prostaglandins within inflammatory tissue which sensitise nerve endings and produce vasodilatation causing pain and swelling.

Disease suppression

Despite the presence of joint damage on the radiographs it is important to prevent disease progression using a disease modifying agent (DMARD). Their precise mechanisms of action are not known but are thought to involve the suppression of pathways of immunological activation including the following:

- Inhibition of lymphocyte activity

- Inhibition of macrophage/monocyte activity

- Inhibition of production / action of pro inflammatory cytokines.

Occupational therapy and physiotherapy: This aspect of therapy should not be underestimated. A full assessment will allow the identification of problems faced by the patient at home. A range of appliances is available to ease daily living for patients with RA.

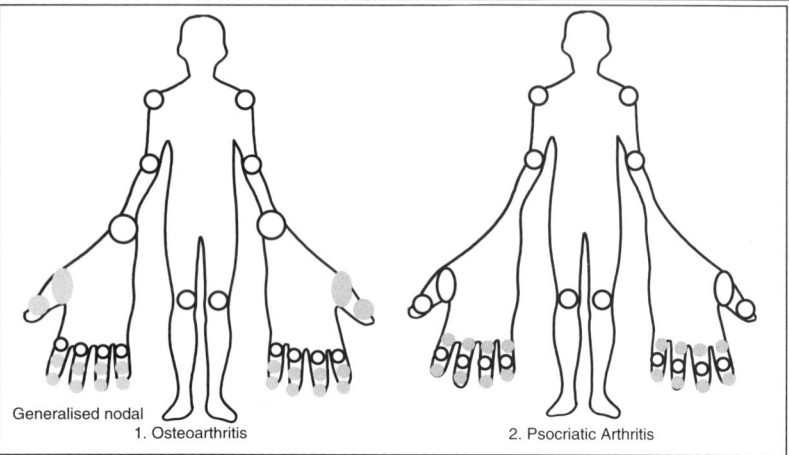

Generalised nodal

1. Osteoarthritis

2. Psocriatic Arthritis

Figure 4: Hand joint involvement in rheumatic diseases

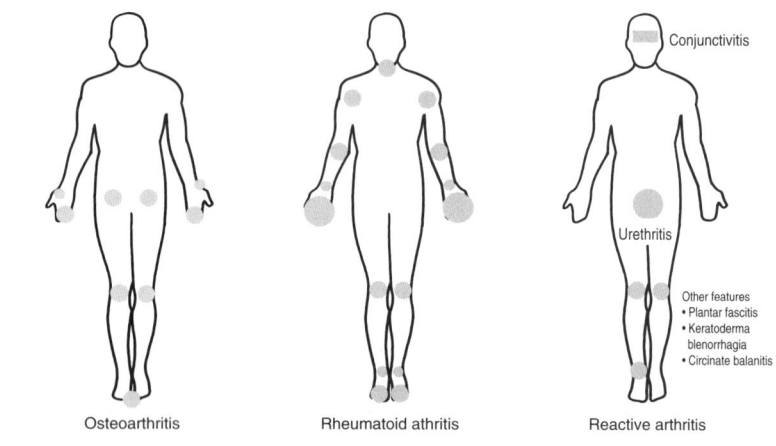

Conjunctivitis

Urethritis

Other features
• Plantar fascitis
• Keratoderma
 blenorrhagia
• Circinate balanitis

Osteoarthritis

Rheumatoid athritis

Reactive arthritis

Figure 5: Joint involvement in rheumatoid arthritis, osteoarthritis and reactive arthritis

CASE 2

Sue, a 25-year-old teacher, and her husband attend your clinic one morning. They have been trying to start a family for the past two years without success. Sue did become pregnant 12 months ago but had a miscarriage at eight weeks. Her past medical history includes a pulmonary embolus at the age of 21.

Physical examination was normal with the exception of this rash on her legs.

The following investigations were performed:

Full Blood Count

Haemoglobin	14.5 g/dL
White blood count	8×10^9/L
Platelet count	70×10^9/L

Clotting Studies

Prothrombin time	15 seconds
	(normal 15 seconds)
Partial thromboplastin time	70 seconds
	(normal 45 seconds)

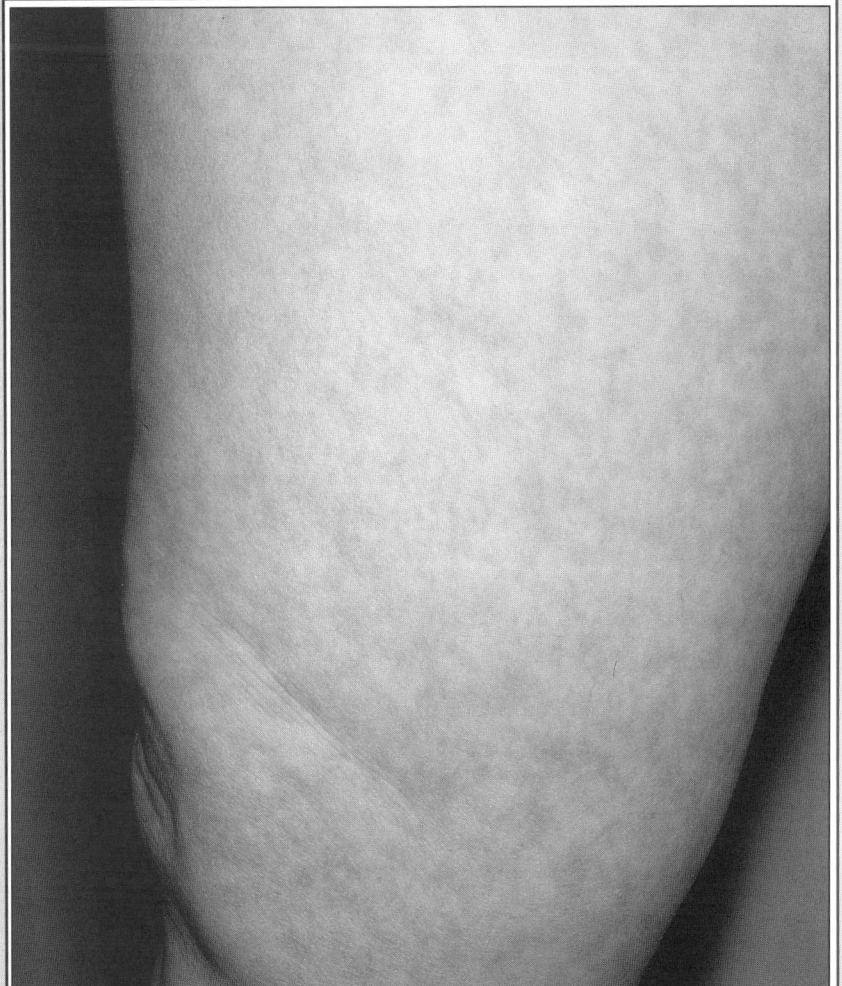

Photograph of right leg

Renal function	Normal
Liver function	Normal
Thyroid function	Normal

What is the name of the rash illustrated?

What do the investigations show?

What is the likely diagnosis?

What treatment (if any) is indicated?

Answer to Case 2

The rash illustrated is livedo reticularis. The reddish blue lattice pattern is due to cyanosis of the skin as a consequence of stasis in the capillaries furthest from their arterial supply. This is an important diagnosis to make because it is associated with a number of underlying diseases. These are listed below.

CONDITIONS ASSOCIATED WITH LIVEDO RETICULARIS	
Physiological	Cutis Marmorata
Vessel wall disease	Atherosclerosis
	Connective tissue disease
	Antiphospholipid syndrome
	SLE
	Polyarthritis
Hyperviscosity states	Polycythaemia
	Thrombocythaemia
	Macroglobulinaemia
Cryopathies	Cryoglobulinaemia
	Cold agglutinins
Congenital	
Idiopathic	

The investigations show a low platelet count and a prolonged APTT. These abnormalities, associated with the clinical features of the patient, give a likely diagnosis of the antiphospholipid syndrome.

The antiphospholipid syndrome is an autoimmune condition characterised by the presence of autoantibodies with affinity for membrane phospholipids.

Antibodies directed against phospholipids predispose to the development of recurrent venous and arterial thrombosis. The complications of this are listed below.

THROMBOTIC COMPLICATIONS OF THE ANTI PHOSPHOLIPID SYNDROME	
Site of Thrombosis	**Complications**
Hepatic	Budd-Chiari Syndrome
	Hepatic Infarction
Adrenal	Addison's Disease
Pulmonary	Thromboembolic Pulmonary Hypertension
Cerebral	Cognitive Impairment
	Movement Disorders, eg Chorea
	Epilepsy
	Migraine
	Transverse Myelitis
Cardiac	Cardiomyopathy
	Valvular Disorders
Renal	Thrombotic Microangiopathy
Dermatological	Livedo Reticularis
	Chronic Leg Ulceration

Antibodies directed against phospholipid in platelet membranes impair their function and result in a higher clearance rate and decreased numbers. Finally, antiphospholipid antibodies interfere with the reagent used in the laboratory to measure the APPT and so produce a prolonged time. Accordingly, the syndrome is characterised by recurrent thrombosis but the prolonged APPT can be misinterpreted as suggesting that the patient has a bleeding tendency.

The diagnosis can be confirmed by measuring the level of

anti-phospholipid antibodies present. In addition, because the syndrome can be associated with SLE, antinuclear and double stranded DNA antibodies should be checked.

The optimal treatment of this condition remains controversial. For patients who have had an episode of thrombosis and have significantly elevated titres of anti-phospholipid antibodies, the recommended treatment is long term anticoagulation with warfarin to maintain an INR of 3-3.5. In a young woman without a previous thrombosis, it would be appropriate to treat her initially with an anti-platelet agent such as aspirin. If she had a thrombotic episode, formal anticoagulation with warfarin would be the first preferred treatment.

CASE 3

John, a 24-year-old labourer, consulted you with low back pain. He described episodes of severe pain and stiffness at the base of his spine radiating into his buttocks. The pain woke him at night and he found that walking about the house helped to relieve the pain. He was very concerned about the symptoms because he had to take two weeks off work.

On examination there was limitation of lumbar spine movement in all directions.

An X-ray of his lumbar spine was arranged and is shown here.

What abnormalities does it show?

What other conditions is this associated with?

What is the appropriate treatment?

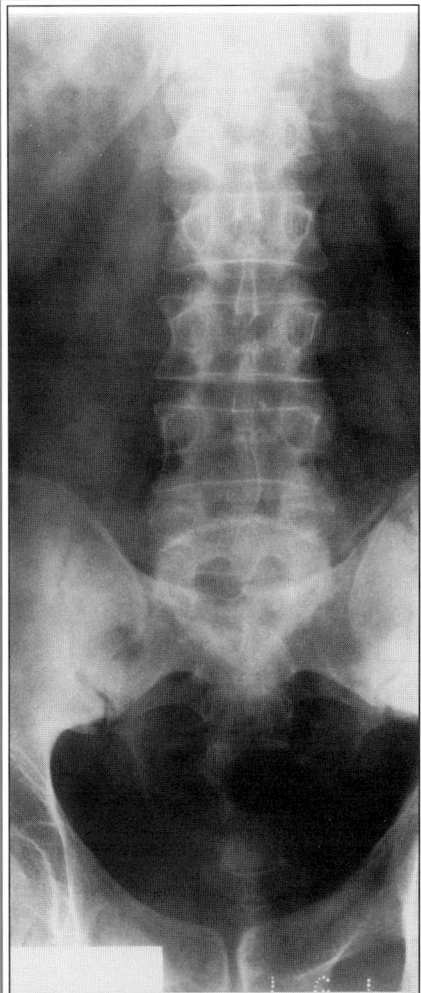

X-ray of lumbar spine and sacroiliac joints

Answer to Case 3

The X-ray shows bilateral sclerosis and erosions on both sides of the articular margin of the sacroiliac joints (SIJ). These changes are typical of sacroiliitis. A CT scan of the SIJ gives a clearer picture as shown here.

Sacroiliitis is a feature of the following conditions:

♦ Ankylosing spondylitis

♦ Colitis associated spondylitis

♦ Reiter's Syndrome

♦ Psoriatic spondylitis.

The conditions are sometimes described collectively as the seronegative (RF negative) spondyloarthropathies. These conditions normally involve the spine and the large joints in an asymmetrical manner. In addition, inflammation of the specialised junction between tendon and bone (enthesitis) is a common feature and causes the symptoms of Achilles tendonitis and plantar fasciitis.

Finally, it is interesting to note that these conditions are associated with the major histocompatability class 1 antigen HLA B27 with varying degrees of association: 90 per cent in ankylosing spondylitis, 60 per cent psoriatic spondylitis and Reiter's Disease. However this is not required to make the diagnosis.

The management principles are to suppress pain and inflammation with NSAIDs and to institute a regular exercise programme in order to maintain spinal flexibility and extension during inflammatory episodes as the tendency is for ankylosis to fix the spine in a flexed position.

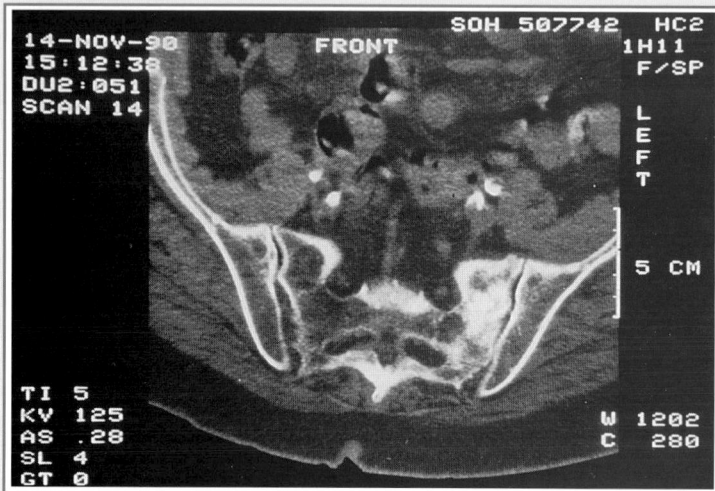

CT scan of sacroiliac joints
There is marked sclerosis of the left sacroiliac joint

CASE 4

Anne, a 55-year-old woman has taken indomethacin for more than two years to treat the pain in her left shoulder. Recently she complained of increasing shortness of breath and constant fatigue. She has not experienced any dyspeptic symptoms.

The results of a full blood count are shown below.

Haemoglobin	8.2×10^9 g/dL
MCV	75 fl
White blood count	4×10^9/L
Platelet count	670×10^9/L
ESR	70mm/hour

A barium meal is organised. This is shown opposite.

What is the likely diagnosis?

Why are her platelet count and ESR elevated?

What measures can be employed to reduce the risk of this complication?

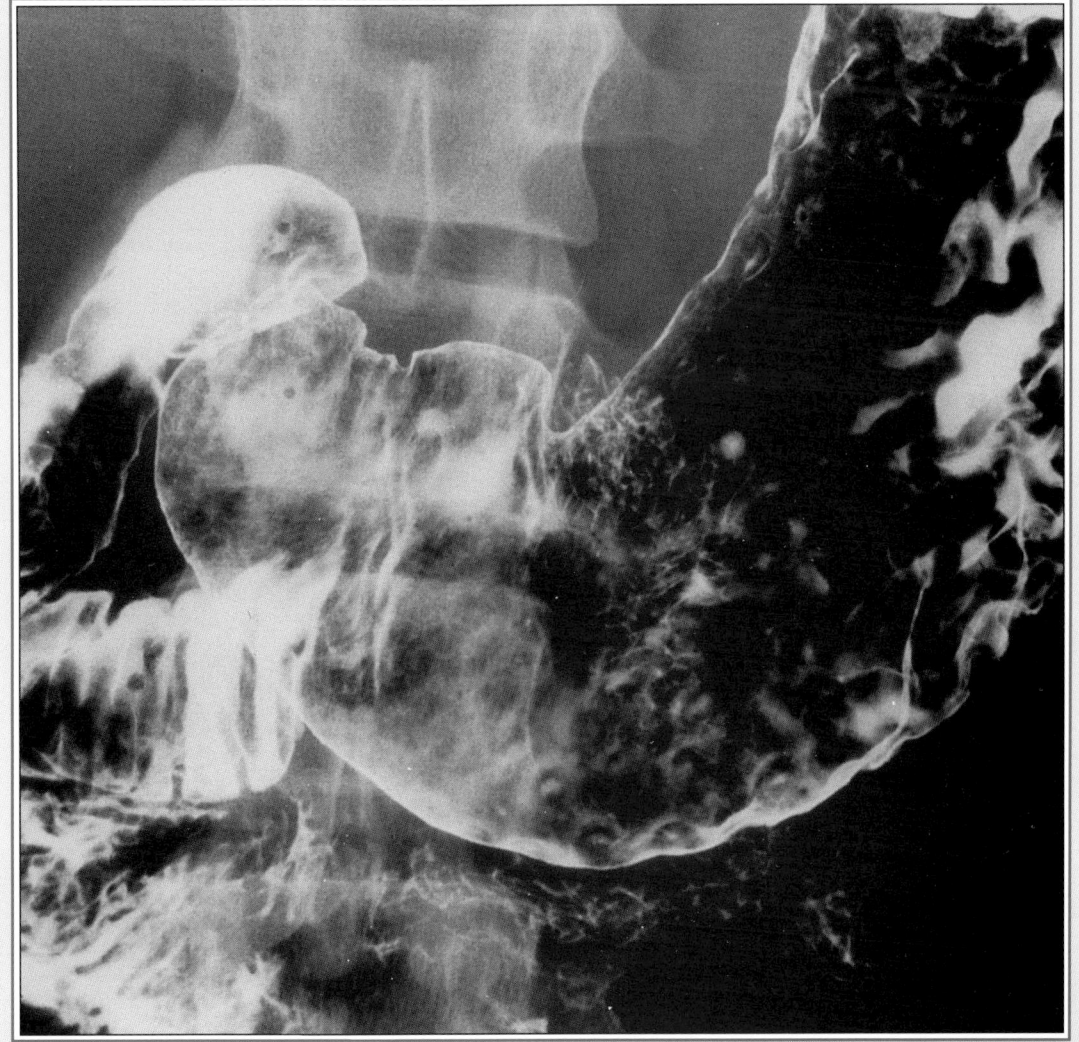

Answer to Case 4

The figure overleaf shows an X-ray of barium meal showing multiple erosions with typical appearance of contrast spot of barium surrounded by lucent rim of oedema.

The most likely diagnosis is NSAID induced gastric erosions causing asymptomatic chronic blood loss and an iron deficiency anaemia. The barium meal demonstrates the characteristic pattern of mucosal ulceration seen in this condition. This is often not associated with any clinical symptoms.

Her elevated platelet count is probably a physiological response to reduce the extent of her bleeding. The ESR is elevated because she is anaemic.

The risk of NSAID induced upper gastrointestinal bleeding can be reduced if the following points are considered:

♦ Does the patient need NSAID therapy? Would simple analgesia with aspirin be sufficient?

♦ Does the patient have risk factors for NSAID induced gastropathy? For example; extreme old age, previous peptic ulcer disease, current steroid therapy

♦ If an NSAID is needed, choose one with a favourable adverse effect profile

♦ Use the minimum dose needed to achieve symptom control

♦ If the patient requires NSAID therapy but is at risk of toxicity, a less toxic NSAID used or a gastroprotective agent, for example misoprostol, could be administered prophylactically.

CASE 5

John, a 40-year-old businessman, attended the emergency department. He had been feeling unwell for the past eight weeks with severe malaise, fevers and dramatic weight loss. Suddenly, while at work, he had developed an acute episode of shortness of breath. He also mentioned that his calf muscles were painful and that his left foot seemed to drag when he walked.

On examination he looked unwell. His vital signs showed a temperature of 39°C, heart rate 120 beats per minute and blood pressure 160/100 mmHg. He had a skin rash which consisted of multiple raised tender red papules. It is shown opposite.

His chest and abdominal examination was normal. His calf muscles were tender to palpation and he was unable to dorsiflex his right foot.

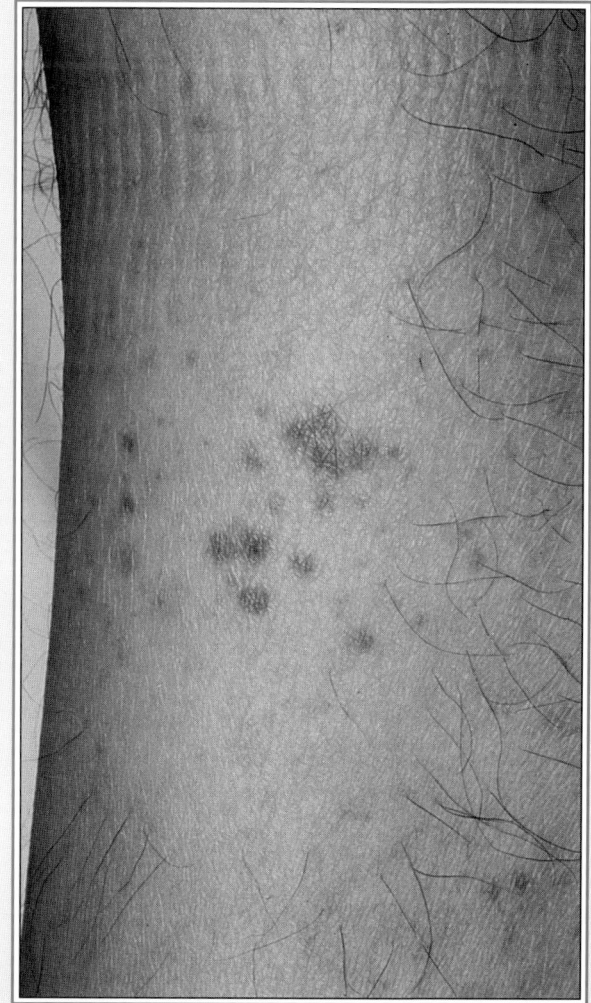

Skin rash

The following investigations were performed:

Full blood Count

Haemoglobin	10 g/dL
White blood cell count	32×10^9/L
Platelet count	900×10^9/L
ESR	120 mm/hour

Renal function

Sodium	140mmol/L
Potassium	5mmol/L
Urea	12mmol/L
Creatinine	154mmol/L

Urinalysis

Protein	+++
Blood	+++

Profuse red cell casts present

Immunology

Rheumatoid factor	Negative
CRP	180 mg/l

What is the differential diagnosis?

What investigations should you perform?

Answer to Case 5

John was clearly unwell with fevers, malaise, a purpuric rash and evidence of a right foot drop. Investigations showed anaemia and a raised white cell and platelet count. In addition, he had a marked acute phase response and evidence of renal impairment.

The most likely diagnosis is a vasculitis but both infection and occult malignancy need to be excluded.

The following investigations are indicated:

♦ Cultures of blood, urine and sputum

♦ Chest X-ray

♦ Echocardiogram

♦ Autoantibody screen including ANCA

♦ Immunoglobulins

♦ Complement

♦ Renal biopsy.

The investigations performed showed that he was positive for pANCA. This is a marker for systemic vasculitis and this was the diagnosis in this case (see Table). It is important to perform a renal biopsy to determine if there is renal involvement present as this will be a major determinant of the type of treatment indicated.

The systemic vasculitides are a group of uncommon conditions which produce inflammation of blood vessels. Since each organ in the body is dependent on an adequate blood supply for normal function they produce symptoms in many body systems.

The diagnosis is made by the combination of clinical features, serological investigations and characteristic histology on tissue biopsy of affected organs, eg renal biopsy.

Systemic vasculitis is a serious condition with a high risk of mortality and requires urgent immunosupressant therapy. Currently the treatment of choice is intermittent intravenous pulse therapy using cyclophosphamide and methylprednisolone.

Anti neutrophil cytoplasmic antibody

Anti neutrophil cytoplasmic antibodies have been used increasingly to help diagnose and monitor the response to therapy in the systemic vasculitides. These antibodies are directed against specific intra cellular components of the neutrophil and may be involved in the pathogenesis of these conditions. There are two major classes of antibodies that have been recognised.

pANCA. This antibody is directed against a myeloperoxidase enzyme within the cell. It is used as a marker for microscopic polyarteritis, but it occurs in a number of other necrotising vasculitides.

cANCA. This antibody is directed against serine proteinase 3 within the cell. It is a specific for Wegener's Granulomatosis.

CASE 6

Tracy, a 20-year-old girl, attended the emergency department of her local hospital with recurrent episodes of anterior chest pain over the last three days.

The pain was not related to exertion but became worse when she took a deep breath in, moved around or leaned forward.

On direct questioning she mentioned that she had been feeling tired and unwell in recent weeks. She had also noted that her hair was falling out and on a recent holiday abroad she had developed a facial rash.

The facial rash is shown. Cardiovascular examination of her chest was normal although it was difficult to hear her heart sounds. There was no evidence of a pleural rub.

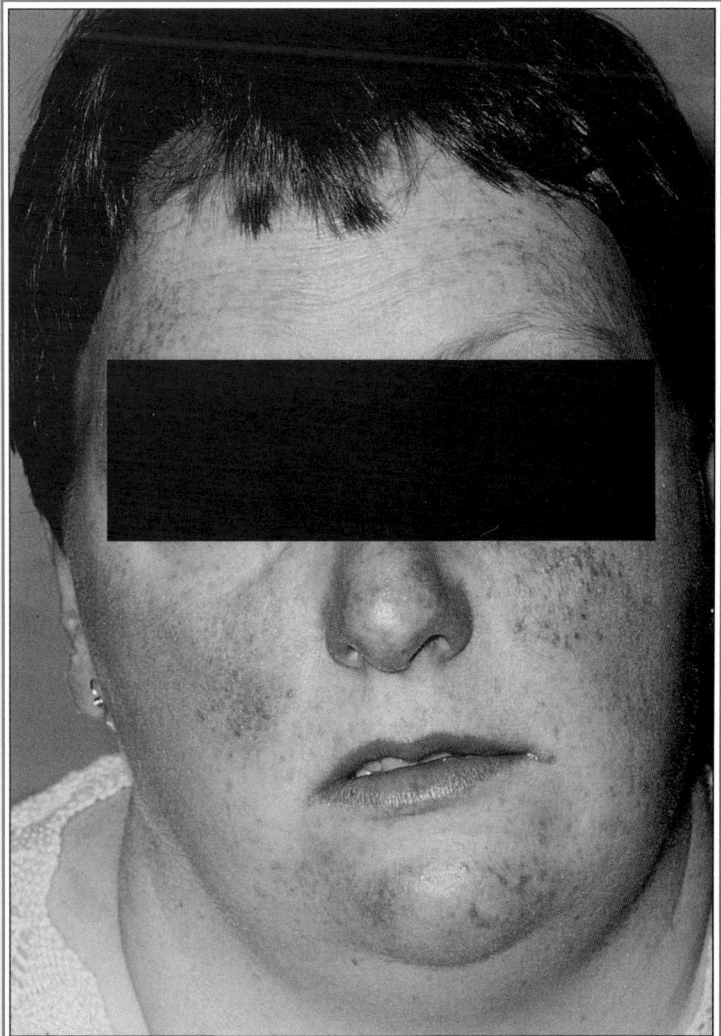

The following investigations were performed:

Full blood count	Haemoglobin	12 g/dL
	White cell count	2.5x10⁹/L
	Platelet count	75x10⁹/L
	ESR	123mm/hour
	CRP	5
Urinalysis	Protein	+++
	Blood	+++
Urea and electrolytes		Normal
Liver function tests		Normal
VQ scan		Normal
Echocardiogram		See opposite

What is the likely diagnosis?

Which further investigations are needed?

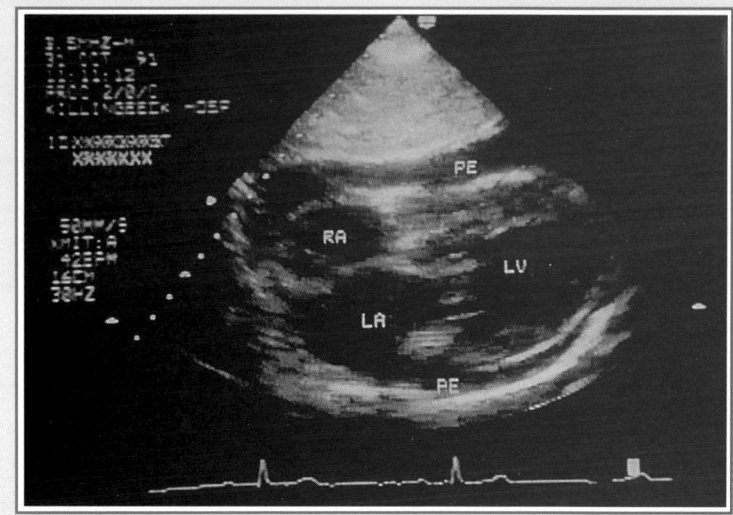

Echocardiogram

Answer to Case 6

The likely diagnosis is systemic lupus erythematosus (SLE) with the classical butterfly rash, alopecia, pericarditis with a pericardial effusion and renal involvement. The low lymphocyte and platelet count and raised ESR are features of active lupus. The abnormal urinalysis indicates renal involvement.

The following investigations are indicated:
Serological investigations to confirm the diagnosis of SLE -

◆ ANA, dsDNA, complement, immunoglobulins

◆ Echocardiogram

◆ Renal biopsy.

The ANA is a sensitive marker for SLE as it is positive in over 95 per cent of patients, but it is not specific as it is positive in a number of other inflammatory disorders.

Double stranded DNA is a highly specific marker of SLE but is present in only 60-75 per cent of cases. dsDNA is thought to play a role in the pathogenesis of SLE and is therefore used as one of the markers of disease activity. A high dsDNA and a fall in complement levels indicate active disease (however a consistently low level of C4 is usually due to a null allele).

An interesting feature of SLE is that the CRP in general is not elevated in active disease, without tissue damage, but will be in the presence of a bacterial infection.

Renal involvement is a common and potentially serious complication of SLE. It needs to be investigated fully because therapy can make a profound difference on long term renal function.

SLE is a multisystem inflammatory disorder with periods of relapse and remission. It characteristically affects young (15-40) women (9F:1M) and presents with a combination of general symptoms plus photosensitivity, rash, Raynaud's Syndrome, polyarthralgia, alopecia, serositis and renal involvement. However it is the renal and cerebral involvement that are responsible for the major morbidity and mortality in SLE.

The commonest manifestations are:

Systemic symptoms: severe lethargy and malaise, moderate weight loss and fever.

Skin rashes: erythematous / papular / urticarial / livedo reticularis. The classical butterfly distribution with involvement over the bridge of the nose and cheeks is very characteristic. Digital abnormalities such as periungal erythema, nailfold capillary dilation or nailfold vasculitis are common. **Photosensitivity** is a characteristic feature.

Raynaud's syndrome: is common but it is usually mild and it may precede the other manifestations of SLE by a number of years.

Alopecia: may be diffuse or patchy and is often a useful guide to disease activity, although it must be remembered that steroids, particularly a fall in dose, can cause hair loss.

Mouth ulcers: these are common in active disease.

Locomotor system: arthralgia or a nondestructive arthritis, frequently including the small joints, is very common.

Pulmonary manifestations: pleurisy and pleural effusions are common. A restrictive lung defect is less common. Pneumonitis and the Shrinking Lung Syndrome (due to vasculitis involving the phrenic nerve), are rare complications.

Cardiovascular manifestations: pericarditis and pericardial effusion are common. Conduction defects, cardiomyopathy and noninfective endocarditis (Libman Sachs endocarditis) are uncommon.

Renal manifestations: proteinuria, nephrotic syndrome and microhaematuria are the commonest manifestations. Diffuse or focal proliferative and sometimes membranous glomerulonephritis are seen on biopsy.

Neurological manifestations: psychosis, CVA, fits, cranial nerve palsies, aseptic meningitis and peripheral neuropathy.

Lymphadenopathy: this is a feature of active disease.

Management of SLE

Because of the variety of organs involved, the management of SLE patients in the past involved many different specialities. It is now apparent that patients are best served by specialist lupus clinics with ready access to all the relevant specialities.

Arthritis, arthralgia and myalgia are the most common manifestations of SLE and are treated with NSAIDs. If this is not effective antimalarials are often of benefit but are slow to act.

Weight loss and fatigue require corticosteroid treatment. Steroid responsive aspects of the disease are shown in the table below.

STEROIDS USE AND SERIOUS DISEASE	
Steriod responsive	**Steroid non-responsive**
Dermatitis	Thrombosis
Polyarthritis	Renal damage
Serositis	Hypertension
Vasculitis	Steroid induced psychosis
Haematological	Infection
Glomerulonephritis	
Myelopathy	

Immunosuppressive therapy using azathioprine and cyclophosphamide is required for life threatening manifestations. Azathioprine is, in general, used for maintenance of remission and can allow reduction of steriod dosage. Cyclophosphamide is used in life threatening conditions (vasculitis, renal disease and severe thrombocytopenia/cytopenia).

Other therapies:

The majority of patients with SLE are photosensitive. These patients should minimise their exposure by wearing clothing and sun screens.

Patients with thrombotic episodes should receive anticoagulants. All patients should have regular blood pressure monitoring and control if needed. Poor control of blood pressure aggravates and maintains renal disease.

CASE 7

This is a series of X-rays which illustrates different aspects of a particular form of arthritis.

Describe the abnormalities shown.

What is the most likely diagnosis?

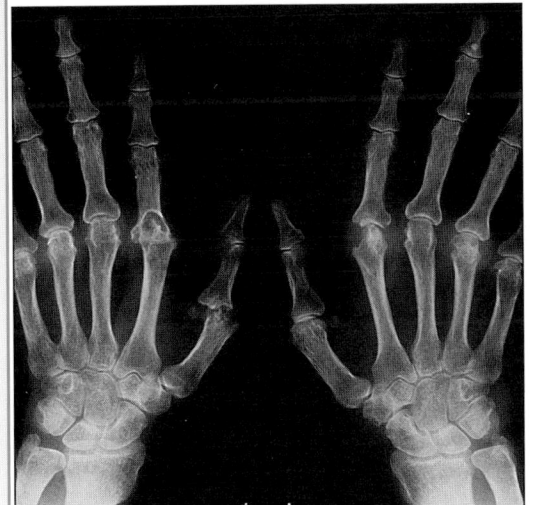

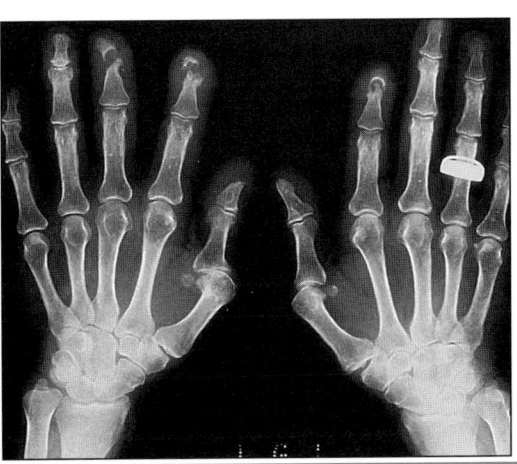

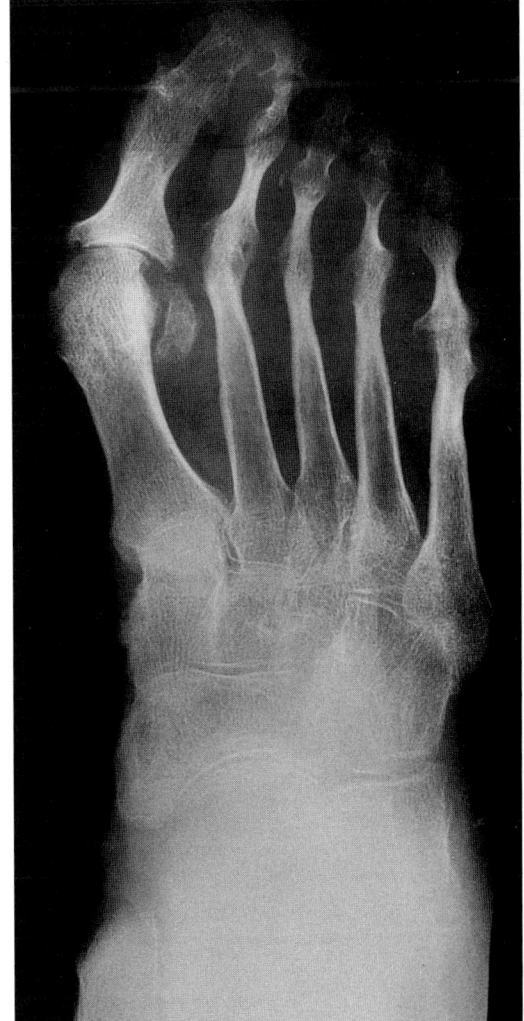

Answer to Case 7

The X-rays show various aspects of psoriatic arthritis. Asymmetrical involvement of the MTP and DIP joints, DIP joint disease with joint destruction and osteolysis, Bone ankylosis of the MTP and an erosion of the first MTP joint.

Psoriasis is a common skin condition. About five per cent of patients with psoriasis develop an associated arthropathy. In adults the psoriatic rash precedes the development of arthritis in about 90 per cent of cases and there is an equal sex incidence. The activity of the arthritis does not usually correlate with the extent of the psoriasis.

There are a number of characteristic radiological features of psoriatic arthritis which help to distinguish it from similar arthritidies. Classically, the joint involvement is oligoarticular and asymmetrical. The erosions affect the marginal areas first, thereby forming a 'pencil in a cup' appearance. The bone mineralisation is well maintained except during an acute exacerbation. A tendency to new bone formation results in spontaneous intrarticular ankylosis, particularly involving the interphalangeal joints and a whiskered appearance around erosions and at the phalangeal tufts. Inflammatory enthesopathies are very common especially involving the ischial tuberosities and calcaneus. Marked periostial reactions are also common.

There are five classical types of arthritis associated with psoriasis:

◆ Asymmetrical oligoarthritis. This usually involves the small joints of the hand and feet and is associated with 'sausage digits'. It may also involve other joints such as the knee, hip, ankle or wrist.

◆ DIP involvement associated with nail dystrophy in the affected fingers. The nails may be pitted or show onycholysis.

◆ A rheumatoid type. This may be clinically indistinguishable from RA but it is rheumatoid factor negative.

◆ Ankylosing Spondylitis type. In these cases about 60 per cent of the patients are HLA B27 positive. Characteristically the spondylitis is segmental, asymmetrical and involves the thoracolumbar area first and has predominant cervical involvement. Paravertebral calcification in the segment involved is characteristic. Sacroiliitis is often unilateral and asymmetrical. Enthesopathies are common especially involving the ischial tuberosities and the calcaneus.

◆ Arthritis mutilans. This is a very destructive form of arthritis. There is resorption of bone resulting in telescoping of the fingers known as 'main en forgette'.

Broadly speaking, the aspects of treatment are similar to that described for RA. They consists of:

◆ Symptomatic relief using NSAIDs.

◆ Disease modifying therapy. It is important to suppress the disease activity to prevent its progression. The preferred DMARDs are, in order of toxicity, methotrexate, cyclosporin and sulphasalazine .

◆ Physiotherapy/occupational therapy. This is an important aspect of treatment to maintain mobility and functional ability.

CASE 8

Dot is an 80-year-old lady who has been unable to lift up her left arm to brush her hair or hang out the wash without getting severe pain in her left shoulder. She's had a number of similar episodes before but this time her shoulder has become progressively stiff.

She was referred to the Rheumatology Department by her GP. There she was seen by the Registrar who ordered an X-ray of her shoulder.

Can you describe the abnormalities demonstrated ?

What is the diagnosis and the most suitable treatment ?

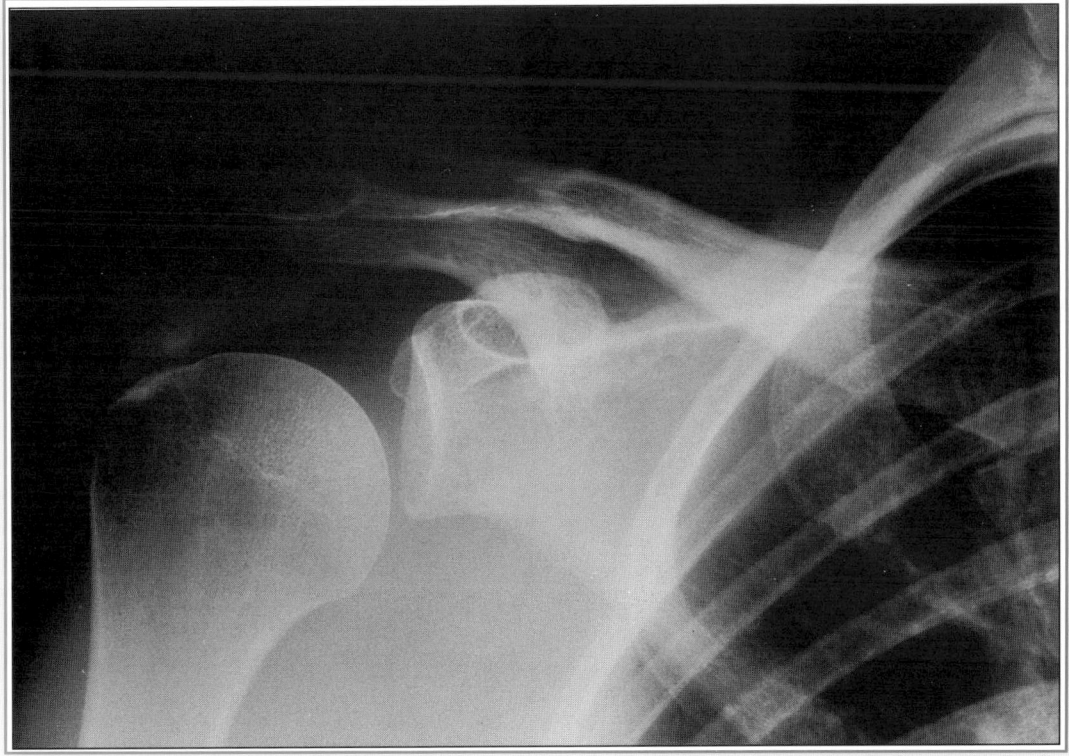

X-ray of right shoulder

Answer to Case 8

The X-ray shows calcification of the suprascapular tendon close to its insertion into the humerus as it inserts in the humeral head (indicating degenerative changes). The patient gave a history of recurrent episodes of shoulder pain in keeping with acute episodes of calcific tendonitis. Now she has developed early adhesive capsulitis.

The Rotator Cuff

The supraspinatus tendons of the supraspinatus, infraspinatus, subscapularis and teres minor muscles are fused to the underlying joint capsule of the shoulder joint and form the rotator cuff. The supraspinatous muscle originates in the supraspinatous fossa of the scapula. It then passes through a narrow area between the coracoid process below and the acromioclavicular joint above, before inserting into the greater tuberosity of the humerus as part of the rotator cuff expansion. Its function is to adhere the humeral head in the glenoid fossa in the early part of abduction performed by the deltoid muscle.

The supraspinatus tendon can become inflamed as it passes through the narrow space between the acromioclavicular joint and the coracoid process. The patient complains of pain at the top of the shoulder on active abduction of the arm between 30 to 60 degrees. On examination there is tenderness over the tip of the acromion. The symptoms are often referred to as a painful arc syndrome.

The aim of treatment is to prevent the development of a frozen shoulder. This is best prevented by relieving the pain in the shoulder which allows the patient to use the joint normally again. The mainstay of treatment is NSAIDs, subacrominal intra articular steroid injections, suprascapular nerve blocks and active physiotherapy.

CASE 9

A middle aged lady was referred to emergency with severe central chest pain. The pain she described was not related to exercise but occurred worst at night and when lying flat.

Photographs of her face and of one of her fingers is shown. She had fine inspiratory crackles at the bases of her lungs.

Her ECG is normal. The chest X-ray shows increased interstitial markings in the lower zones.

What is the likely diagnosis?

What investigations are appropriate?

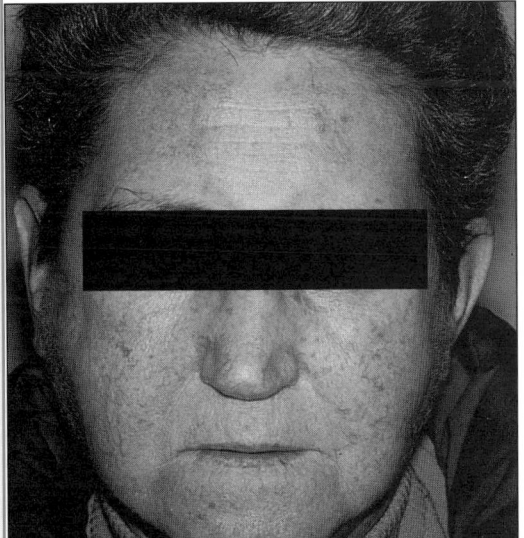

Figure 1: Facial appearance of patient

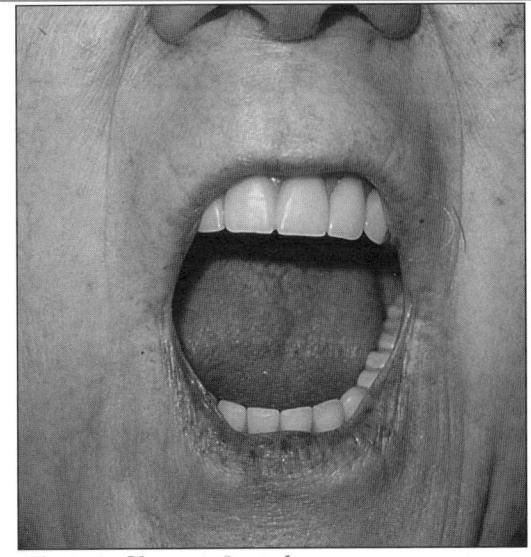

Figure 2: Close up of mouth

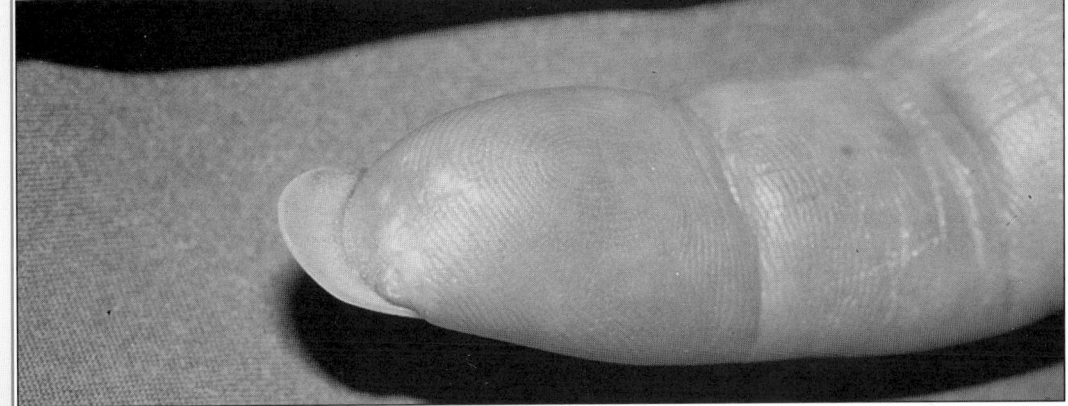

Figure 3: Finger of patient

Answer to Case 9

The diagnosis is diffuse systemic sclerosis. This is an autoimmune condition characterised by progressive sclerosis of blood vessels, skin and internal organs. This is in contrast to localised scleroderma in which there are similar clinical and histopathological changes in the skin but systemic features are absent.

Appropriate further investigations include FBC, ESR, CRP, autoantibody screen including anticentromere antibody, barium swallow and lung function tests.

Systemic sclerosis

The condition is characterised by the following features:

Skin: The changes in the hands illustrate the progressive pathological changes that take place. There are three phases: an inflammatory phase, a dermal fibrosis phase and an atrophic phase. During the inflammatory phase the fingers become swollen and sausage like from a combination of nonpitting oedema of the skin, synovitis and tenosynovitis. Pathologically, this is due to inflammation in the skin and subcutaneous tissues with lymphocytic perivascular infiltrates and swelling and degeneration of collagen fibres. Following this, the skin gradually becomes thickened, waxy and tethered. This is due to the increased formation of dermal collagen by the fibroblasts and the gradual obliteration of the blood vessels due to intimal proliferation and the dilation of the remaining ones resulting in telangiectasia. Finally, the skin becomes atrophic and appears thin with areas of pigmentation and vitiligo. There is also loss of the subcutaneous fat and resorption of the distal phalanges.

Skin changes start in the hands, then progress to involve the face, forearms and chest. The tight tethered skin results in flexion contractures in the fingers and a beaked nose and microstomia with circumoral puckering of the surrounding skin.

Raynaud's phenomenon: This is almost an invariable feature. It frequently precedes the other features of SS. It is often severe and causes digital infarcts and ulceration.

Gastointestinal disease: The progressive sclerosis causes mobility problems and dilation. Oesophageal involvement is very common and causes dysphagia, reflux oesophagitis and aspiration pneumonia. In the small bowel, the atony and dilation can cause abdominal cramps, or a stagnant loop type syndrome with bacterial overgrowth and malabsorption. Similar changes in the large bowel result in constipation and mechanical obstruction. The formation of wide mouthed pseudodiverticulae is very characteristic but is usually asymptomatic.

Pulmonary involvement: Progressive basal fibrosis is an early and common feature and leads to increasing respiratory failure. Pulmonary hypertension is a late feature, primarily of the localised (CREST) variant due to involvement of the pulmonary arteries.

Peripheral arthritis: If there is an arthritis it is usually mild and involves the small joints of the hands. It is also common to find leathery crepitus over the wrist or patella due to tenosynovitis.

Myopathy: There may be either a myositis or a myopathy.

This is easily missed. Shoulder girdle weakness may become very severe. A commonly recognised variant of the disease is the CREST syndrome. This is characterised by subcutaneous calcinosis, Raynaud's phenomenon, oesophageal dysmotility, sclerodactyly and telangiectasia.

Investigations: FBC, this may show the anaemia of chronic disease, ESR is often elevated.

Immunological investigations: 70 per cent of patients are ANA positive. 30 per cent of patients are RF positive. The SCL-70 antibody is associated with progressive systemic disease. The anti-centromere antibody is associated with the CREST variant of the disease.

On examination of her hands, the skin is thick, waxy and tethered causing loss of skin creases and claw hand deformity. There is sclerodactyly due to the loss of finger pulp, nailfold telangiectasia, subcutaneous calcification and areas of ulceration at the fingertips. (See Figure 3). On her face, the tight skin causes microstomia and a beaked nose, she has multiple telangiectasia (Figure 2) and will have severe Raynaud's Syndrome. She will probably have problems due to oesophageal dysmotility, basal lung fibrosis and cardiac arrhythmias. Mortality from SS is from respiratory failure, pulmonary hypertension, malignant hypertension, renal failure or arrhythmias.

Treatment: There is no standard disease 'modifying' treatment for the underlying disease process. The aim of treatment is to provide symptomatic benefit for individual problems.

Raynaud's phenomenon: Vasospasm of the digital arteries can be improved by arteriolar vasodilators such as nifedipine. If it is severe, some patients require prostaglandin infusions.

In addition, a cervical sympathectomy can be effective - a simple prophylaxis against the condition is heated gloves.

Pulmonary fibrosis: There is no definitive treatment, though in selected cases immunosuppressive treatment with cyclophosphamide and prednisolone, is beneficial.

Oesophageal dysmotility and oesophagitis: Simple advice such as taking regular small meals, sitting upright, antacids, and omeprazole can all be effective.

Gut dysmotility and malabsorption:
Renal involvement: endarteritis of renal arterioles can result in progressive renal failure and malignant hypertension. This is a serious life-threatening complication. It is important to control the blood pressure to prevent strokes and reduce the rate of renal deterioration.

CASE 10

Selwyn returned from a wonderful break in the West Indies. The sun, sand and women were all fantastic! He spent all day lying on the beach and all night partying in clubs.

Six weeks after returning home his right knee and left ankle and heel became swollen and painful. He also noticed a rash and peeling of the skin on the soles of his feet.

What is the diagnosis ?

What investigations are indicated?

How should he be treated ?

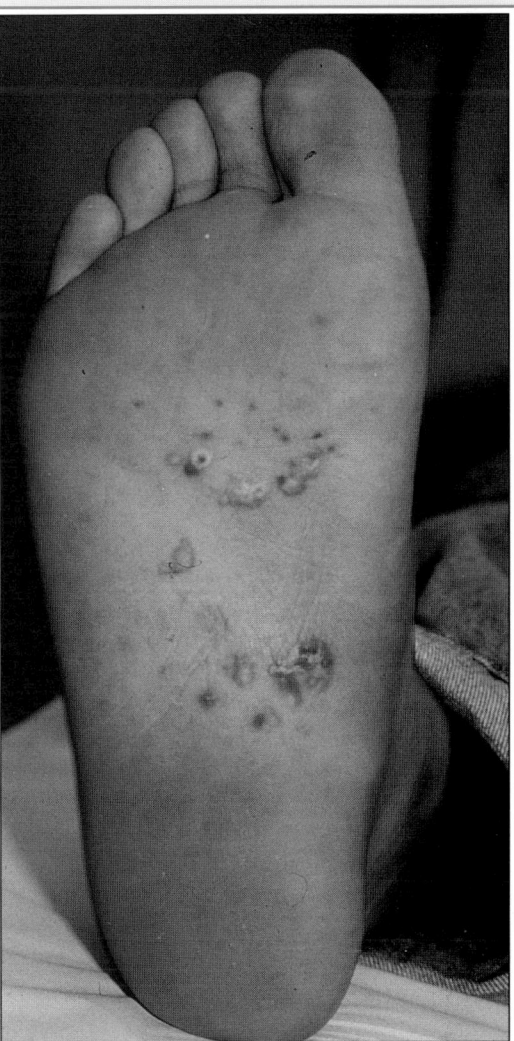

Answer to Case 10

The symptoms described are suggestive of a reactive arthritis. This is an inflammatory reactive arthritis which occurs following either an episode of urethritis or gastroenteritis. The triad of arthritis, urethritis and conjunctivitis is often referred to as Reiter's Syndrome.

The infection appears to trigger the onset of symptoms but they may then develop and recur independently of the original stimulus. There is a marked male preponderance (20:1) and increased risk (40 x) in the HLA B27 positive population.

The following infective agents are associated with the condition:

Gastroenteritis	Salmonella
	Shigella
	Campylobacter
	Yersinia
Urethritis	Chlamydia

Selwyn had recently travelled abroad raising the possibility of both travellers' diarrhoea and unprotected sexual intercourse. Clearly both of these possibilities need to be discussed and appropriate samples taken.

The urethritis is usually due to infection with *Chlamydia trachomatis* and it presents about two weeks after intercourse with a clear penile discharge and dysuria. He may also have *Circinate balanitis* which presents as a painless, superficial ulcer surrounded by erythema on the glans.

Up to a month after the episode of urethritis, between one and two per cent of patients develop acute Reiter's Syndrome with oligoarthritis, tenosynovitis, conjunctivitis and keratoderma blenorrhagia. The oligoarthritis predominantly involves the lower limb joints and is asymmetrical. This is frequently accompanied by plantar fasciitis or Achilles tendonitis.

Keratoderma blenorrhagia is an uncommon but highly characteristic rash which usually only occurs on the palms and the soles. It presents as small brown macules which rapidly develop into papules and then sterile pustules, which are similar to pustular psoriasis. This is associated with severe hyperkeratosis which results in intense scaling and loss of the nails. The conjunctivitis may be mild and often goes unnoticed.

Following this, about a third of patients develop spondylarthopathy with recurrent flares. In these circumstances it is appropriate to give a disease modifying agent; sulphasalazine is the agent of choice. The treatment for the urethritis is a two week course of oxytetracycline which may well decrease the severity of the arthritis and the likelihood of recurrent episodes. Reiter's and psoriatic spondylarthopathy are very similar and share radiographical characteristics (see Case 7).

CASE 11

Eric was a professional footballer for many years. Now in his fifties, he suffers with pain in his knees. Here's an X-ray of his right knee.

What does it show?

What conditions predispose to its development?

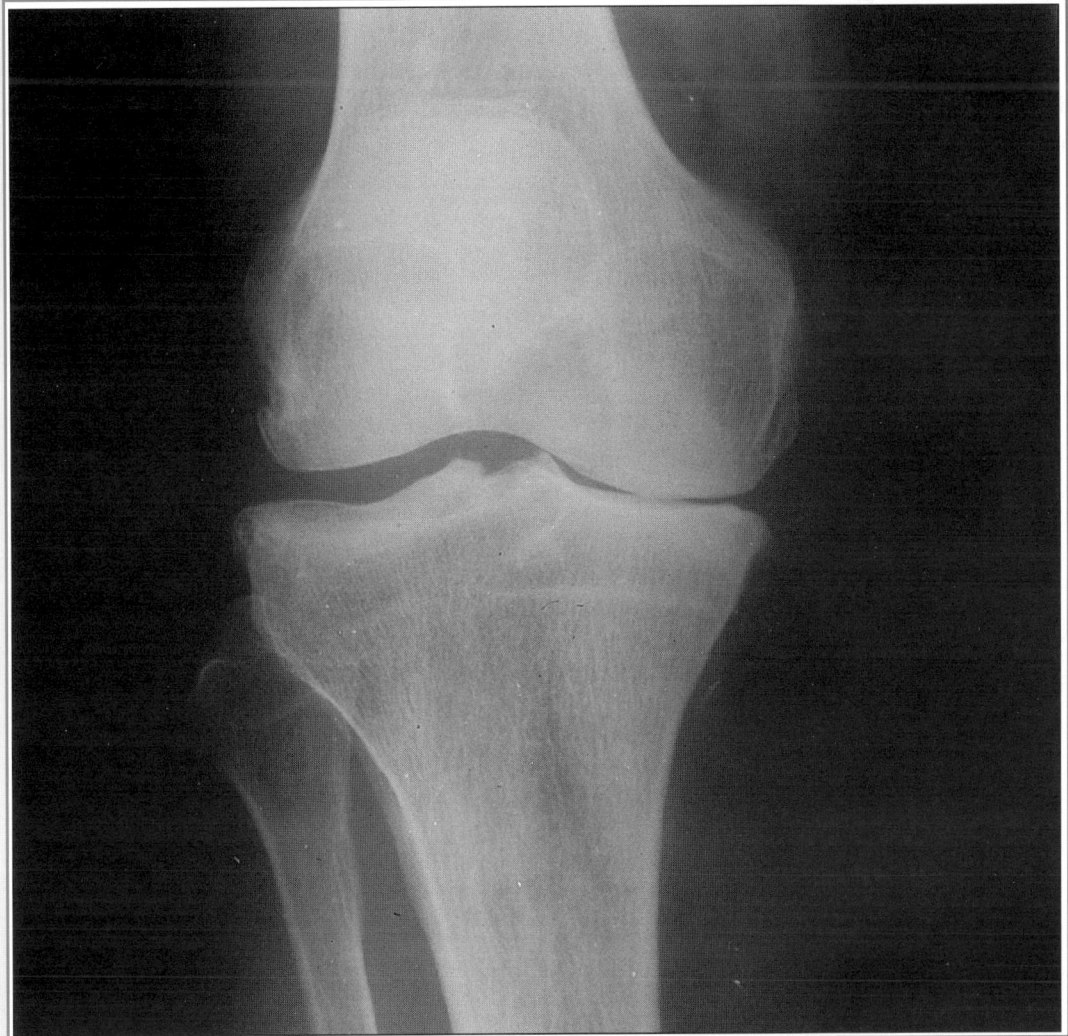

Answer to Case 11

The X-ray shows asymmetrical loss of the joint space and sclerosis of the joint margins due to osteoarthritis affecting the medial compartment of the knee. The knee is a complex joint with three major compartments; the medial and lateral tibiofemoral joint and the patellofemoral joint. Each compartment can be affected, separately or in combination. Isolated medial compartment or medial plus patellofemoral disease are the commonest combinations. In Eric's case this is due to the heavy wear on his knee joint during his football career.

Osteoarthritis is a degenerative condition which affects synovial joints. It can be primary or secondary to an earlier process which has damaged the joint. Its incidence increases with age and commonly affects the cervical and lumbar spine and weight-bearing joints such as the knee and hip. Common causes for secondary osteoarthritis include inflammatory arthritis, heavy wear, eg knee joints in skiers or footballers, neuropathic joints, avascular necrosis, operations such as a meniscectomy, and congenital deformity, eg. a dysplastic hip. Progression is slow and occurs over decades. If progression is more rapid than this, then a vascular abnormality such as avascular necrosis should be considered.

Clinically, patients complain of pain in the affected joint which is worse after use or in the evening and relieved by rest. There may be a short period of early morning stiffness and stiffness after immobility. On examination, if there is an acute flare, the joint will be painful, warm and swollen due to an effusion. Chronically the joint becomes deformed with bony swelling due to the osteophyte formation and there is pain crepitus, and limitation of movement.

Pathologically, the first signs of damage are the appearance of cracks and fissures at the surface of the articular cartilage known as fibrillation. Arthroscopically, it loses its lustre and the surface looks velvety. As the process continues there is patchy loss of the articular cartilage causing exposure of the underlying bone which becomes hardened and eburnated.

Subchondral cysts also develop where synovial fluid is forced into the underlying exposed bone. Bony remodelling results in the development of osteophytes around the articular margins.

Radiologically, these changes are seen as asymmetrical loss of joint space with underlying sclerosis and subchondral cysts.

Primary generalised nodal osteoarthritis

Primary generalised nodal osteoarthritis is an autosomal dominantly inherited condition. It characteristically affects middle aged women and affects the DIP and PIP joints as well as the hips, knees and spine. Heberdens nodes (at the DIP) and Bouchards nodes (at the PIP) initially appear as firm swellings which produce a clear gelatinous material if aspirated. If they are left alone they become bony. First one, then other joints become involved. The onset is therefore described as 'stuttering'. Fortunately good functional ability is maintained in spite of the marked deformity.

Evidence for the systemic nature of this condition comes from the finding that if these patients undergo a medial meniscectomy of the knee, they develop medial compartment osteoarthritis more rapidly than people who do not have the condition.

New developments in OA

OA has been regarded as a degenerative 'wear and tear' condition of articular cartilage. However, there are several pieces of evidence to suggest an inflammatory component to OA: (1) the presence of morning stiffness and a good response to NSAIDs can be taken as evidence of an inflammatory process, (2) using highly specific assays (for C-reactive protein) it is possible to demonstrate an acute phase response in OA and (3) the presence of 'hot' joints using radioisotope scans.

New drugs which combine the properties of a DMARD (for the treatment of RA) and a NSAID have been developed. In clinical studies of OA they have been shown to effectively suppress the acute phase response and disease progression in animal models. If such 'disease modification' can be reproduced in human studies it will represent an important advance in treatment.

CASE 12

Joint replacement (or arthroplasty) has developed into a highly effective treatment for end stage joint disease. However it is associated with a number of complications

What are they?

Which ones are illustrated here?

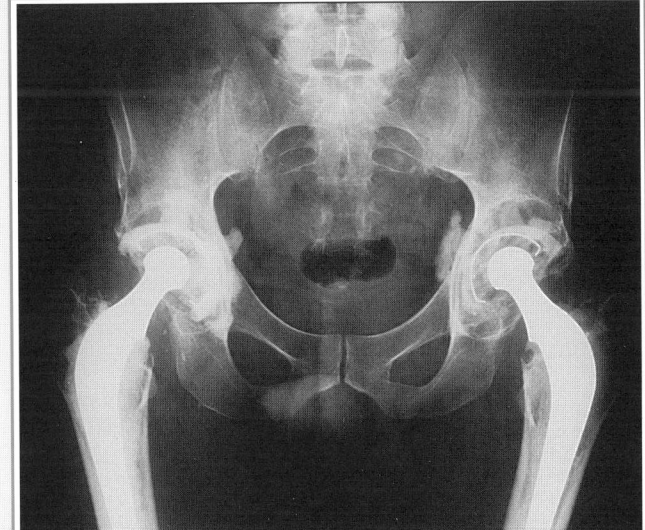

Figure 1

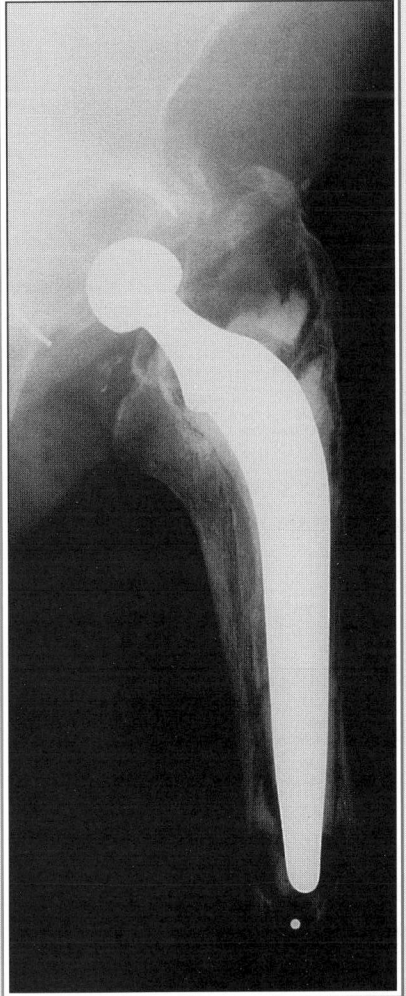

Figure 2

Answer to Case 12

The following complications are seen:

Figure 1 - Loosening of the acetabular component of a total hip replacement. This is more marked on the left.

Figure 2 - Loosening of the femoral stem of a total hip replacement.

Infection: The infection rate after joint replacement has been dramatically decreased over the years by the introduction of prophylactic antibiotics and extreme care over aseptic techniques, including the use of tent or costumes with unidirectional airflow. The expected rate is now as low as one per cent. Early infection is due to airborn contamination of the wound at the time of surgery. Late infection is probably due to haematogenous spread from distant sites within the body. So patients should have prophylactic antibiotics before procedures which cause a bacteraemia such as a dental extraction or a urological procedure.

Osteolysis due to host response to debris: The presence of debris from the procedure including tiny particles of metal, cement and polyethylene all incite a host response. The debris is phagocytosed by macrophages which then become activated and cause osteolysis around the prosthesis which finally leads to loosening.

Heterotopic bone formation: New bone may be progressively laid down around the joint. This leads to limitation of its range of movement. It is thought that local mesenchymal cells are stimulated by the traumatic stimulus at the time of operation to transform into osteoblasts. Certain groups are at a higher risk of this heterotopic bone form, eg ankylosing spondylitis.

Fractures: Fractures can occur in the prosthesis or the surrounding bone. If the prosthetic component in the femoral shaft is stronger than bone, the surrounding bone becomes weaker as it is shielded from the stress it requires to maintain its bone mass.

Dislocation: Dislocation may occur for a number of different reasons. The first, is that the patient attempts to put the joint into a position beyond the range of the prosthetic components. The second, is there may be an imbalance of the surrounding musculature or malpositioning of the components, so that even with use within the normal range, the components dislocate in certain positions.

CASE 13

Bill, a middle aged businessman, has had sinusitis and an intermittent bloody nasal discharge with crusting for the past two years. Recently, he began to feel rather unwell, with a mild fever and a cough productive of white phlegm streaked with blood.

He also developed a pain over the right side of the back of his chest which worsened when he coughed or took a deep breath.

On examination he looked unwell and had a right sided pleural rub.

The following investigations were carried out:

Full Blood Count

Haemoglobin	9.0 g/dL
White cell count	6×10^9/L
Platelet count	400×10^9/L
ESR	99 mm/hour
CRP	230 mg/L
Arterial blood gases pO$_2$	8Kpa
pCO$_2$	3.5Kpa
pH	7.3

Here is his chest X-Ray. What does it show?

What is the most likely diagnosis?

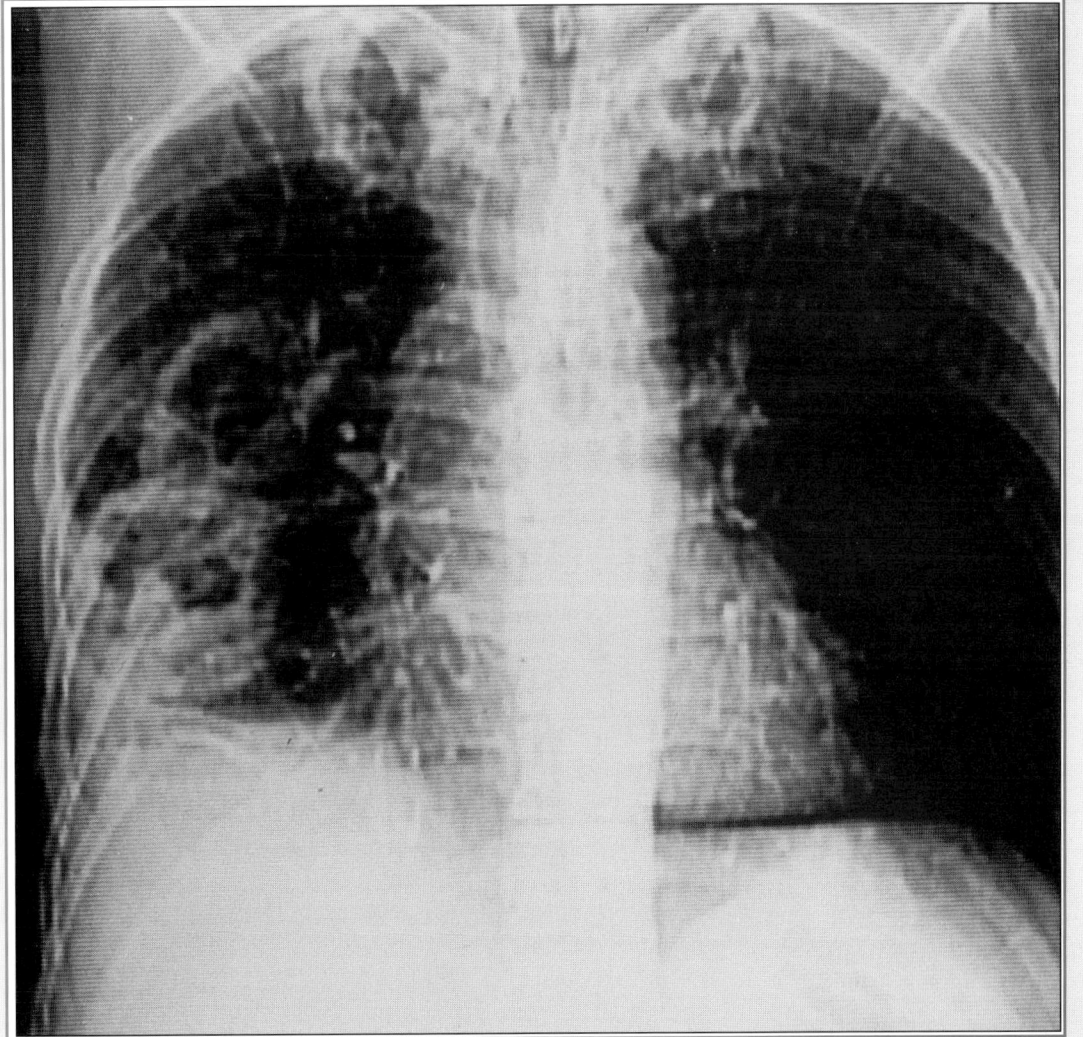

Chest X-ray

Answer to Case 13

The CXR shows multiple large nodules in the right side of his chest.

The clinical picture is suggestive of Wegener's Granulomatosis.

This is a vasculitis which predominantly affects small arteries and is characterised by the formation of necrotising granulomas. The vasculitis most commonly involves the upper and lower respiratory tract and the kidneys (known as limited when latter not involved). It usually affects middle-aged men and is preceded by a prodromal period of malaise, low grade fever, fatigue and marked weight loss.

Upper respiratory involvement includes the nasal passages, sinuses and ears. This can cause nasal stuffiness, a bloody nasal discharge, sinusitis, serous otitis media and deafness. A CT scan of the sinuses is often useful and shows mucosal thickening. Granulomas in the lungs cause pleurisy, dyspnoea and pulmonary haemorrhage. A chest X-ray with multiple large poorly defined opacities in this situation may be either due to pulmonary nodules or haemorrhage. A simple non invasive way to differentiate the two, is to perform a transfer factor which would be raised in pulmonary haemorrhage.

The renal lesion is usually a focal and segmental glomerulonephritis with or without the presence of crescents which can progress rapidly and cause acute renal failure.

It is important to obtain a tissue diagnosis from a biopsy specimen from the kidneys, involved nasal mucosa or lung. Characteristically, the inflammatory markers are raised and there is a neutrophilia, a thrombocytosis and hypergammaglobulinaemia. In Wegener's there is usually a high titre of cANCA.

As with all the vasculitides, there is multisystem involvement including neurological abnormalities such as mononeuritis multiplex, conjunctivitis or scleritis, rashes such as purpura or livedo reticularis and arthralgia.

This is a serious life-threatening condition. It requires intensive immunosupression commonly with pulses of intravenous methyl prednisolone and cyclophosphamide.

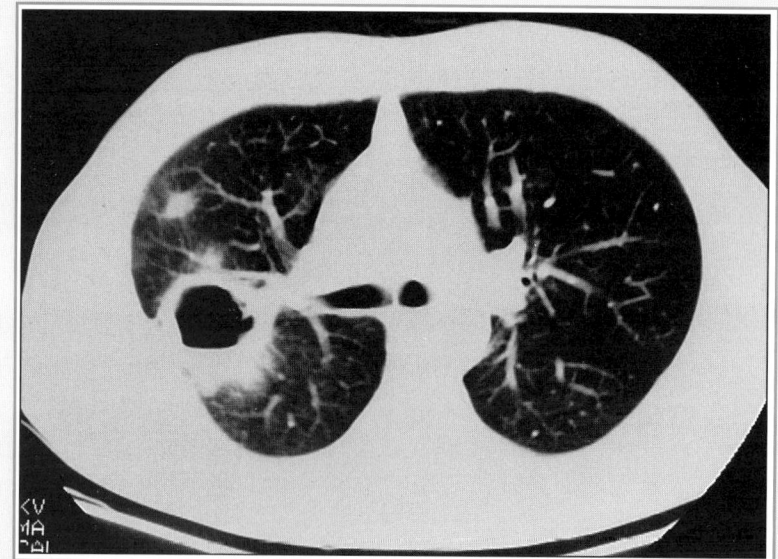

CT scan of chest showing cavitating lesions in the right lung

CASE 14

Annie is the wife of the local bar owner. However, now she is not able to serve behind the bar because of the pain in her right groin. It started gradually a few months ago, but then it only really troubled her at the end of a long shift after she had been standing up for hours.

After a few weeks she visited her GP who ordered an X-ray of her pelvis and hips. This was normal and the doctor reassured her that it would probably settle in a few days. However, it became worse and she was in constant pain. Finally, she was persuaded by her husband to visit her local emergency department. She was seen by the orthopaedic clinician who repeated the X-ray and then ordered an MRI scan.

What are the abnormalities shown on the X-ray and MRI scan?

What are the commonest predisposing factors for this condition?

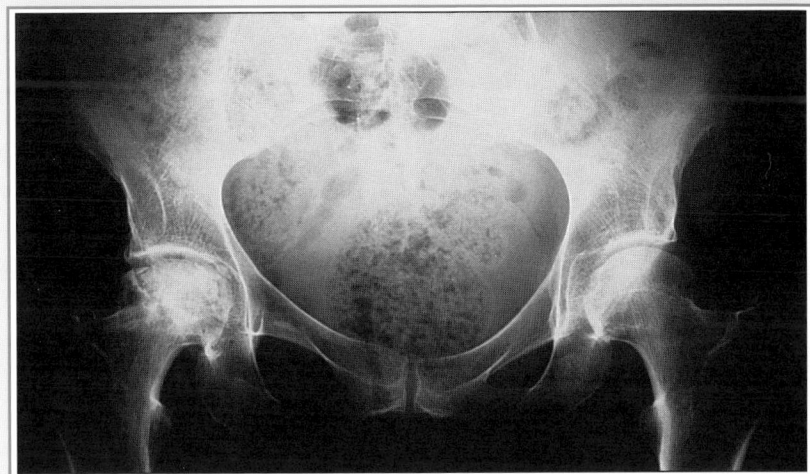

Figure 1: X-ray of pelvis

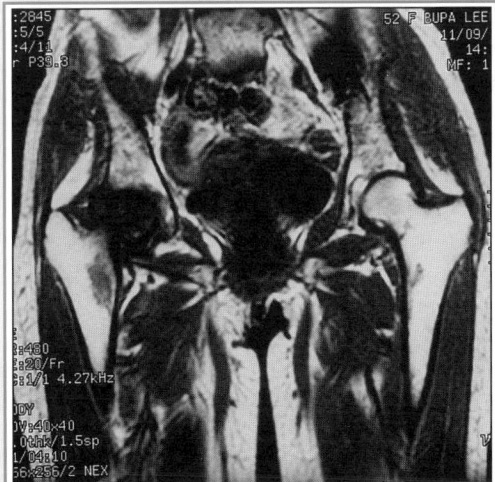

Figure 2: MRI scan of pelvis (coronal section)

Answer to Case 14

Annie has avascular necrosis (AVN) affecting the head of her right femur.

Avascular necrosis occurs when the blood supply to an area of bone is interrupted. The head and distal femur, head of the humerus, the scaphoid, lunate and metatarsal bones are the commonest sites affected. There are multiple predisposing factors but the commonest are fracture or dislocation, high dose steroid usage, chronic alcohol excess, vasculitis or abnormal accumulation of cells within the bone marrow, as in Gaucher's Disease.

Once the blood supply is interrupted, the affected area infarcts and becomes necrotic. Where it abuts normal bone, there is a margin of hyperaemia. It is from behind this that the granulation tissue and then new bone formation extend. Gradually, the whole area becomes sclerotic. However, the affected area is very weak and may well collapse under the strain of normal use, particularly in a weight bearing area such as the femur. This leads to further joint disruption and severe secondary osteoarthritis.

AVN causes an insidious onset of symptoms. Pain is usually the main complaint and it is exacerbated by weight-bearing. However, AVN may be asymptomatic and be an incidental finding on X-ray. Examination of the affected joint is often normal, unless the bone has collapsed, or secondary osteoarthritis has developed causing pain and limitation of movement.

X-ray changes are not apparent for many weeks. The first signs are an area of radiolucency with a sclerotic margin demarcating it from the normal bone. At this stage the joint line is maintained. Later, the whole area becomes sclerotic due to a combination of the laying down of new bone and collapse of the trabeculae (see Figure 1). The crescent sign, which is the radiological hallmark of AVN, is a late feature and is seen as a radioluscent line parallel to the joint line between the sclerotic bone and the normal bone as they separate.

Fortunately, AVN can be detected in its early stages with an MRI scan (the investigation of choice) or a bone scan. A bone scan initally shows a cold spot when the area is necrotic and then a hot spot due to the active process of regeneration. An MRI scan will clearly show up the affected area as a low intensity signal bordered by a high intensity signal.

Initial treatment consists of bed rest to prevent joint loading. In theory, the consequent reduction in joint pressure will increase the chances of the damaged blood supply re-establishing itself. If conservative treatment is not successful, orthopaedic surgery may be required.

Figure 1 shows AVN of the right hip with sclerosis and collapse of femoral head.

Figure 2 shows a low intensity signal from the right femoral head on both T1 and T2 weighted images. This indicates non viable bone.

CASE 15

Brian is a sixty-year-old man who has had seropositive rheumatoid arthritis for 15 years.

He has been treated with intramuscular gold for the last 12 years. Over the last 12 months he has developed progressive dyspnoea and a dry cough. A chest X-ray and pulmonary function tests were performed. The results are shown below.

	Observed (litres)	Expected
FEV1	2	2.5-3.8
FVC	2.5	3.2-5
TLC	4.7	5-7.5
TLco	3.6	7.2-11mM/min/kPa

What abnormalities are shown on the chest X-ray?

What pattern of lung disease do the pulmonary function tests show?

What is the diagnosis?

What treatment options are available?

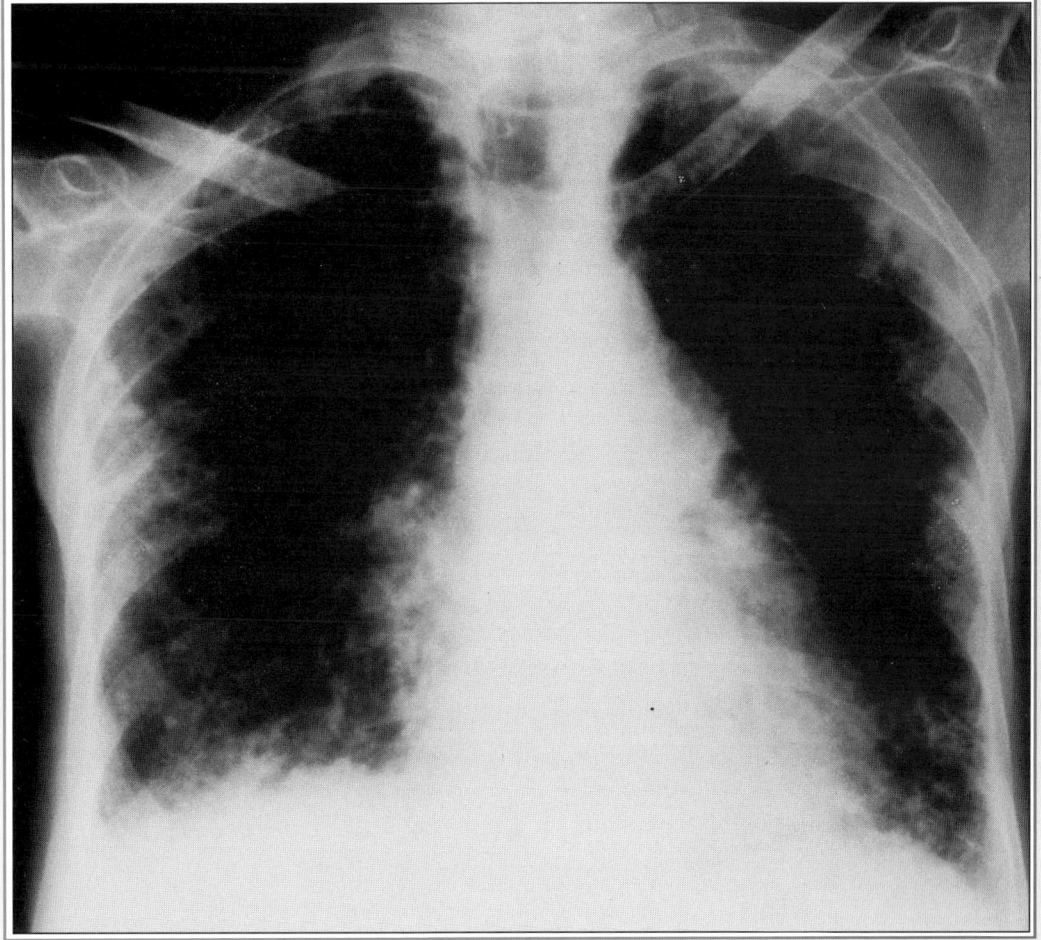

Chest X-ray

Answer to Case 15

The chest X-ray shows widespread interstitial shadowing with honeycomb formation consistent with interstitial fibrosis. The lung function tests demonstrate a restrictive pattern with decrease in lung volumes, an increase in FEV1/FVC ratio and a reduction in gas transfer. This pattern is typical of diffuse pulmonary fibrosis in association with rheumatoid arthritis and is clinically indistinguishable from idiopathic fibrosing alveolitis. It is more common in male rheumatoid patients and smokers.

Treatment is empirical with trials of high dose oral steroids, often in combination with immunosuppressants such as azathioprine or cyclophosphamide. Bronchoalveolar lavage can be useful in predicting the response to steroids as those patients with a predominant lymphocyte excess in the lavage fluid tend to respond better than those with predominant neutrophils.

The possibility of drug induced lung disease should also be considered. Acute pneumonitis associated with gold therapy is well described but whether it contributes to chronic changes is debatable. Most cases of acute pneumonitis reported have occurred within the first year of therapy and around 40 per cent of these have a significant eosinophilia. The outlook for this patient is good. The time course in this patient suggests it is unlikely that gold is implicated.

THE PULMONARY COMPLICATIONS OF RHEUMATOID ARTHRITIS
Diffuse pulmonary fibrosis
Pleural effusion
Parenchymal pulmonary nodules
Caplan's syndrome
Bronchiolitis Obliterans
Isolated pulmonary arteritis

CASE 16

Edith, a sixty-year-old lady presents with a one year history of pain in her hips and pelvis. An X-ray of her pelvis is requested and is shown opposite.

What abnormalities are shown on the X-ray?

What is the differential diagnosis?

What further investigations are indicated?

What is the most likely diagnosis?

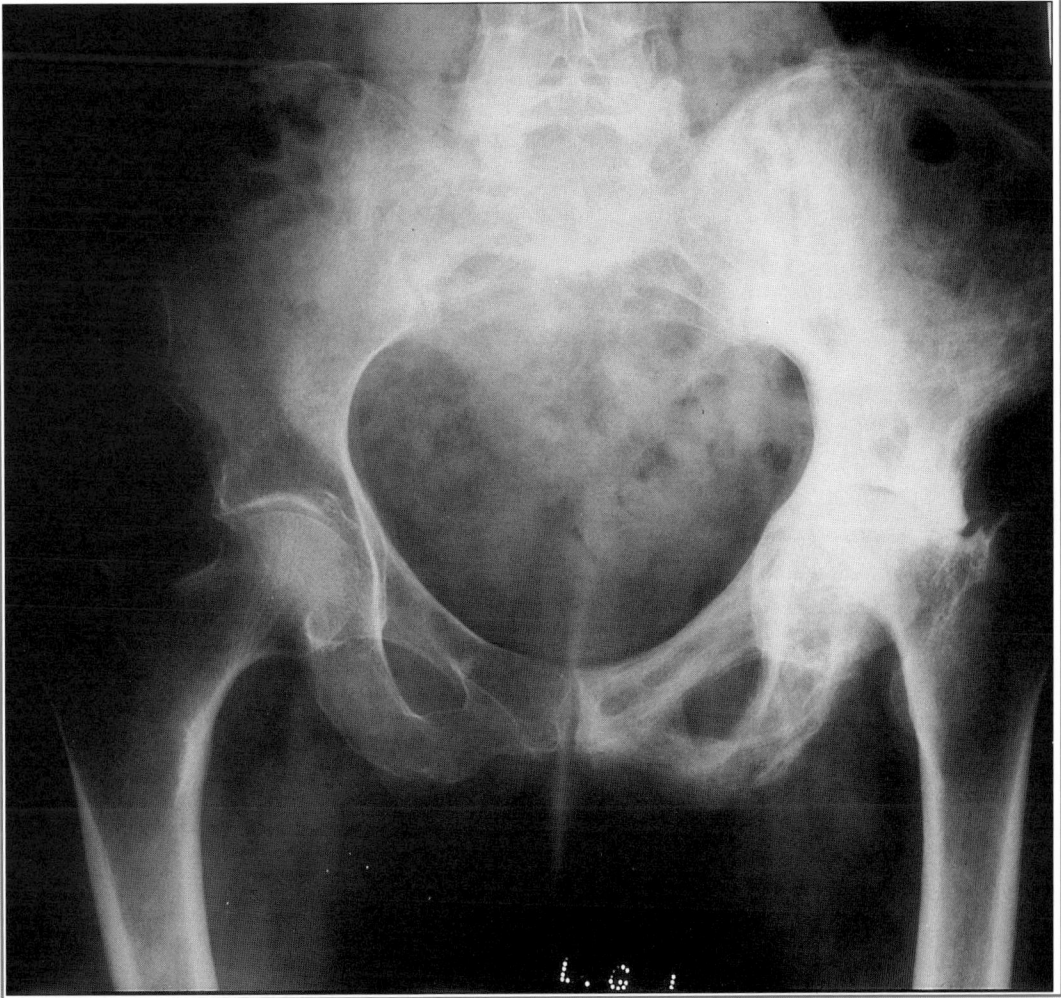

X-ray of pelvis

Answer to Case 16

The main diagnoses to consider are Paget's Disease, sclerotic metastatic disease (eg prostatic carcinoma in a man), lymphoma and haemangioma.

Further investigations which should be performed include bone biochemistry and an isotope bone scan. Most cases of Paget's Disease are associated with an elevation of bone alkaline phosphatase but the serum calcium is usually normal unless the patient is immobilised. Hypercalcaemia would suggest malignancy as a more likely diagnosis. If there is still diagnostic uncertainty the lesion should be biopsied.

Paget's Disease affects around five per cent of the UK population over the age of 55. The cause is unknown although various viral theories have been suggested. Any bone can be affected but lumbar spine and pelvis are the most frequent sites. The disease process involves accelerated bone remodelling with increased osteoclast mediated bone reabsorption followed by compensatory increases in new bone formation. This produces disorganised bone structure, deformity and increased fracture risk. Sarcomatous transformation can occur in pagetic bone producing increasing pain and swelling with X-ray changes of developing osteolysis and bone spiculation.

In this case, the bone scan revealed a further diffuse area of increased uptake in the left hemipelvis and plain X-rays confirmed typical appearances of Paget's Disease.

Paget's Disease is treated symptomatically using simple analgesia, NSAIDs and physical therapy. The development of safer and more effective treatments to suppress the disease process of Paget's Disease has lead to the introduction of such therapy at an earlier stage. These drugs provide effective symptom relief and act to inhibit the activity of osteoclasts. The choice of treatment falls between the bisphosphonates and calcitonin.

Bisphosphonates

These drugs are analogues of pyrophosphate (calcium pyrophosphate is the major mineral in bone) and effectively suppress the disease process. The first generation bisphosphonates could produce a reversible defect on mineralisation, with increased risk of fracture. This was minimised by vitamin D supplementation. More recently developed bisphosphonates appear free of this side effect. Treatment is often given for six months with a three month treatment-free period to permit recovery of the mineralisation defect.

Calcitonin

Subcutaneous or intramuscular calcitonin is a safe effective treatment. A problem which may occur is disease relapse after initial treatment benefit due to down regulation of the calcitonin receptors.

CASE 17

A 50-year-old female presents with progressive bilateral hip discomfort. She has always been supple and was a keen gymnast as a child.

Examination reveals restriction in movement at both hips. The skin is hyperextensible as shown here. She admits to longstanding problems with skin healing and easy bruising.

A pelvic X-ray confirms bilateral hip osteoarthritis.

What is the diagnosis?

What other complications are found in this condition?

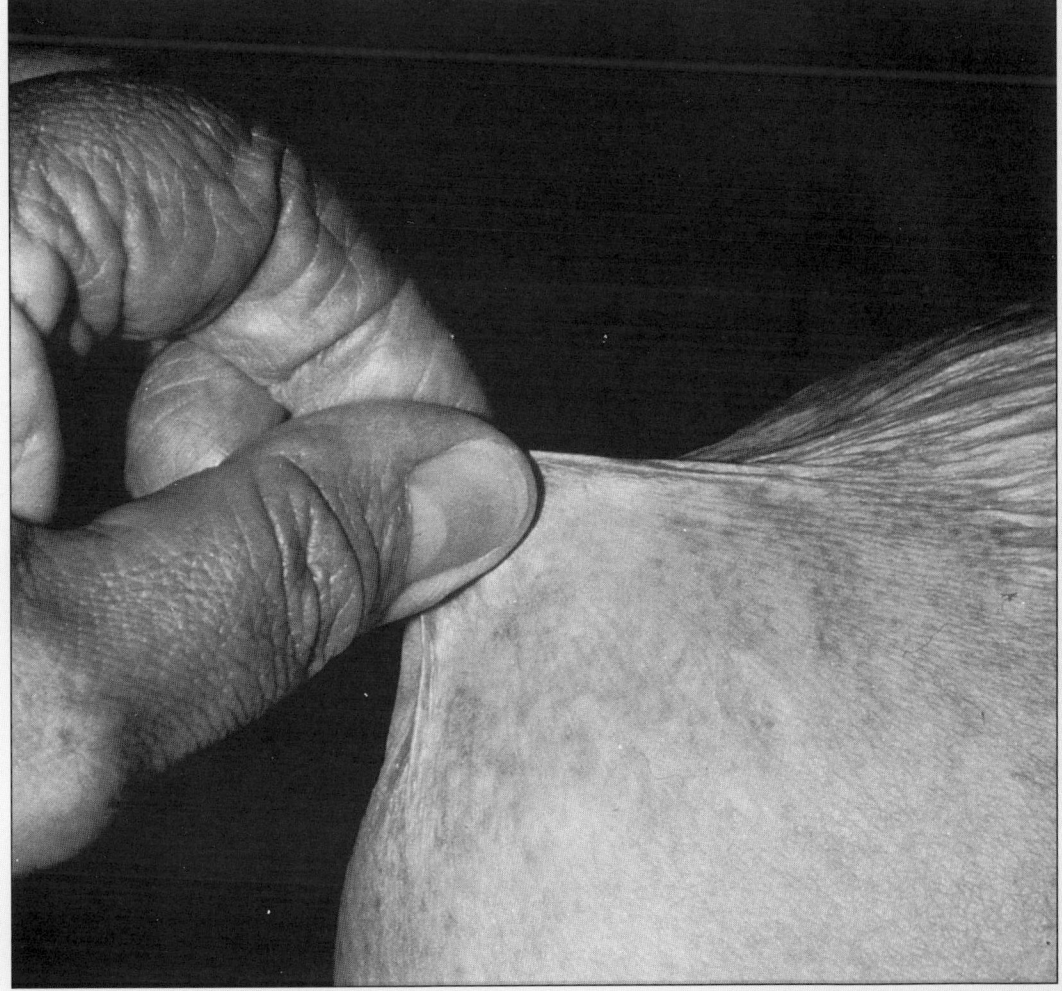

Figure 1: Hyperextensible skin

Answer to Case 17

The photographs show abnormal skin extensibility (Figure 1) and scar formation (Figure 2). These appearances are typical of Ehlers-Danlos Syndrome.

This is an inherited condition affecting connective tissue with abnormalities of the skin, joints and blood vessel walls. Ten subtypes have been identified with variations in clinical features, severity and inheritance pattern. Most are autosomal dominant or X-linked recessive disorders.

Joint involvement includes hypermobility, recurrent dislocations, and in some cases, premature osteoarthritis. Major complications can result from vascular involvement including arterial dissection and rupture. Rupture of the colon and pregnant uterus have also been described. Mitral valve prolapse is a common feature.

These complications are seen predominantly in type IV Ehlers - Danlos Syndrome which is one of the rarer subtypes and is associated with defects in type III collagen synthesis or secretion. Other subtypes are associated with defects in type I collagen, fibronectin and other enzyme deficiencies.

There is no effective treatment for this condition. It is important that a full explanation be given to allow avoidance of situations which place undue stress on the joints.

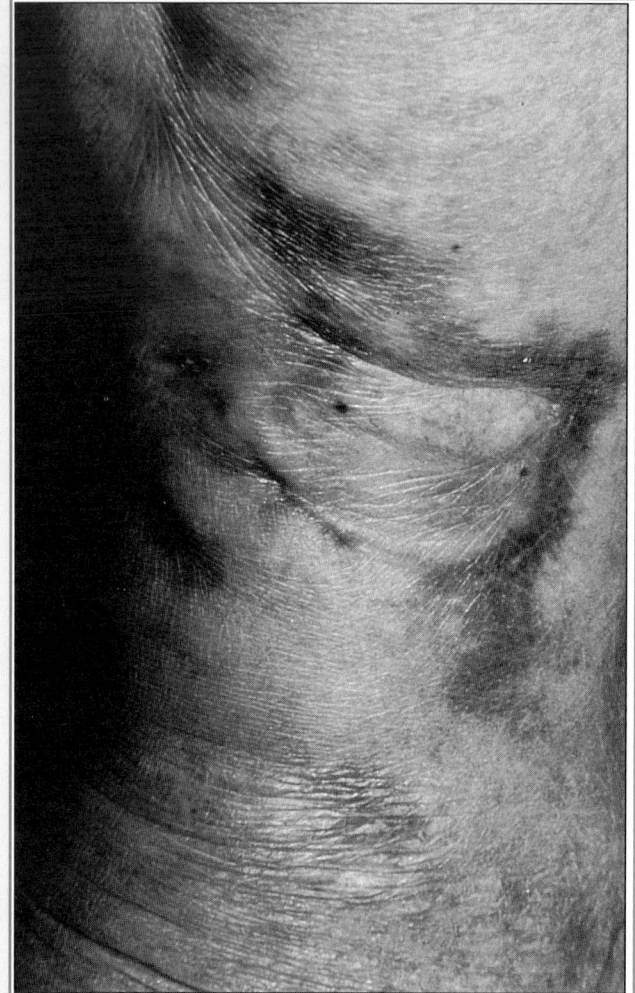

Figure 2

CASE 18

Elaine, a 25-year-old secretary, attended the outpatients' department complaining of cervicobrachial pain. The pain radiated into the lateral side of the forearm and hand. Her symptoms worsened when carrying heavy shopping and she found reaching up with her arms above her head uncomfortable. She also had longstanding symptoms of Raynaud's Syndrome.

On examination, there was a full range of movement in the cervical spine and no abnormality on neurological examination. Examination of the peripheral joints was also normal. Peripheral pulses are easily felt in the resting position but the radial pulse became impalpable when her arm was raised above her head.

Nerve conduction studies were normal.

Her subclavian angiogram is shown.

What is the most likely diagnosis?

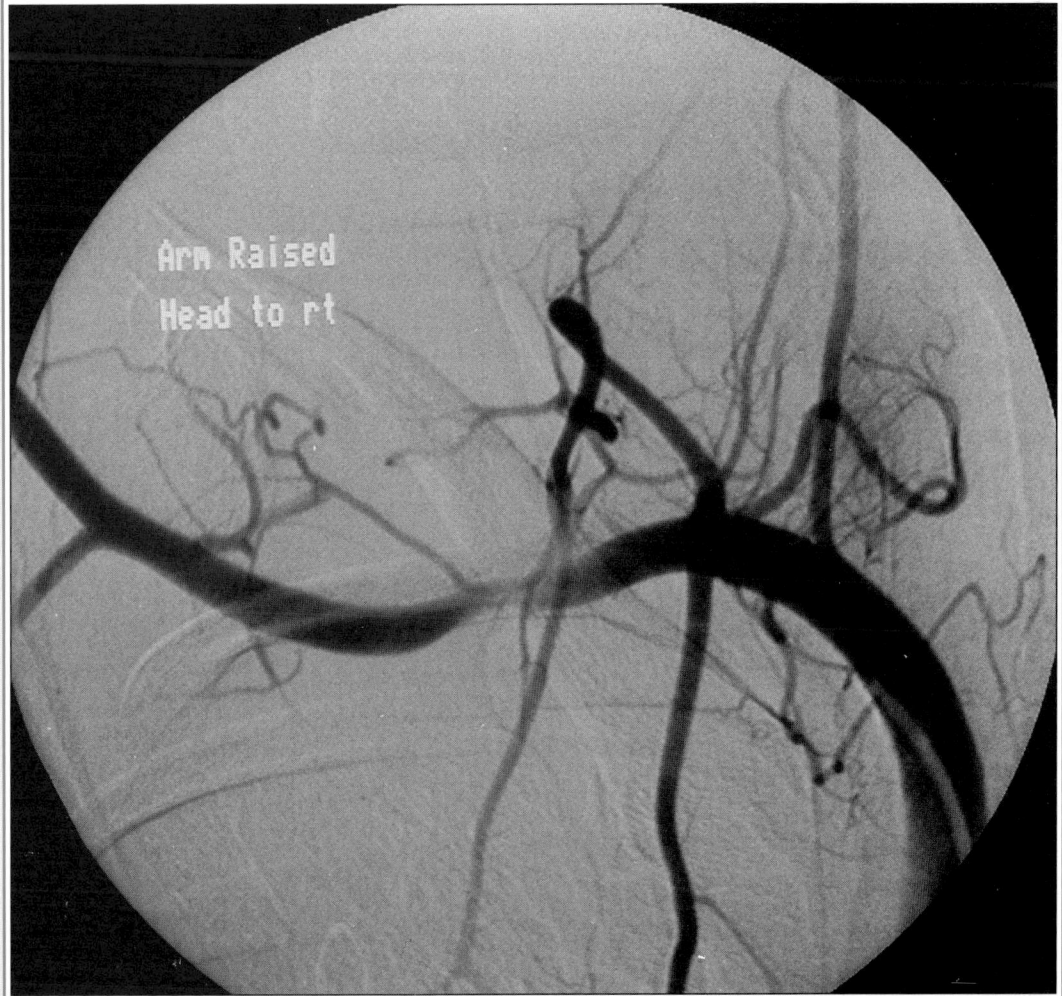

Angiogram of the right subclavian artery

Answer to Case 18

This young lady describes typical symptoms of thoracic outlet syndrome due to compression of the subclavian vessels and the lower trunk of the brachial plexus as they pass through the cervicothoracic outlet.

There are three narrow areas where compression can occur, namely around the scalene triangle, costoclavicular passages and the pectoralis minor attachment to the coracoid process. The narrowing may be associated with a cervical rib, an abnormal first rib or with a fibrous band. In some cases, no structural abnormality can be identified.

Obliteration of the radial or bronchial pulse may be noted, either when the patient takes and holds a full breath with the head tilted back or rotated laterally (Adson's test), or when the arm is abducted and externally rotated while the shoulders are rotated (Wright's manoeuvre). These tests can be positive in thoracic outlet syndromes but are not reliable indicators.

In this case, the angiogram taken with the arm raised and neck rotated shows compression of the subclavian artery as it passes through the costoclavicular passage. Unless there is evidence of neurological deficit or significant vascular insufficiency, management should be conservative. More severe cases should be referred for surgical decompression.

Conservative treatment with shoulder girdle exercises and postural training is all that should be advocated for mild disease but may fail to remove all symptoms. Surgical intervention is often unsuccessful, carries considerable risk and should be avoided except in patients with serious vascular or other complications.

Operations that have been advocated include: resection of the first rib, resection of cervical rib, claviculectomy, scalenectomy with soft tissue release and partial scalenectomy.

CASE 19

Robert is a 20-year-old art and design student living away from home. He has recently begun to feel very tired and has had recurrent mouth ulcers.

He went to see his G.P. because of pains affecting his hands, wrists, feet and knees. He denies any genito-urinary symptoms or gastro-intestinal upset. His past medical history is unremarkable except for the minocycline he has been taking for acne vulgaris for the past 18 months. He has recently changed his sexual partner.

What is your differential diagnosis?

What investigations would you order?

What is your management plan?

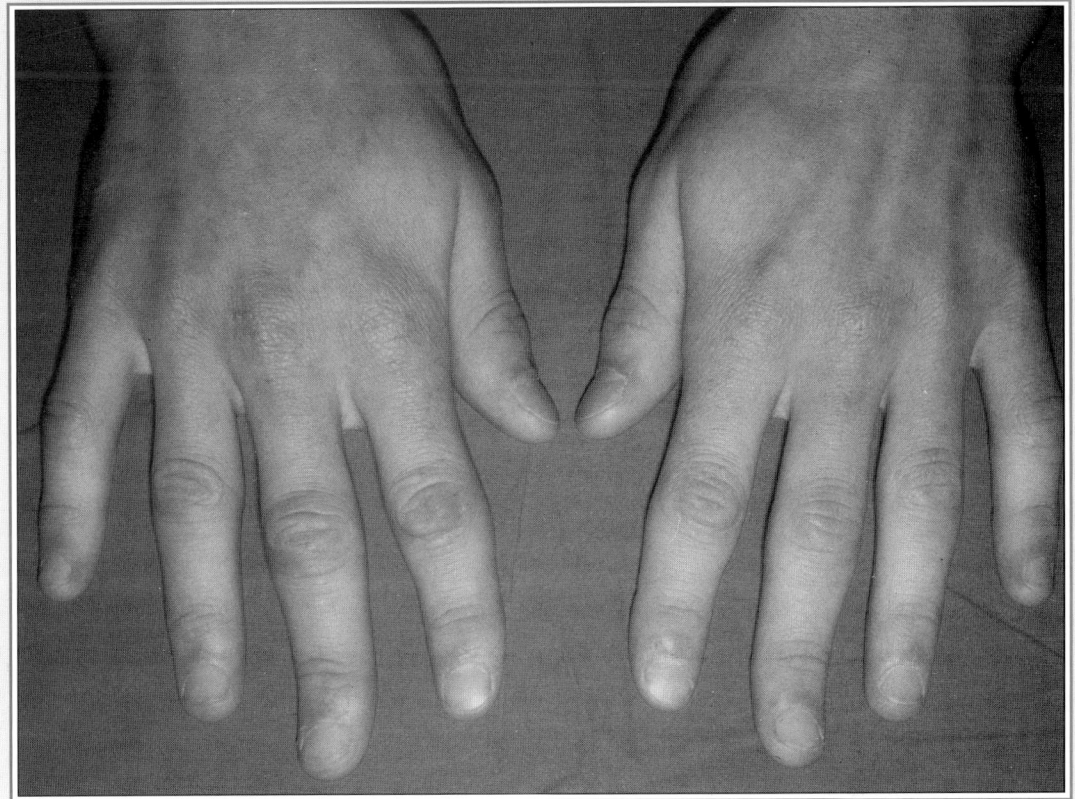

Answer to Case 19

Differential diagnosis:

Drug-induced lupus

Reactive arthritis

Reiter's Syndrome

Behcet's Disease.

Investigations:

Antinuclear antibody

Double stranded DNA binding

Complement (C3, C4) levels

Full blood count

ESR

Chlamydia/Yersinia serological testing.

In this case, Robert has drug-induced lupus.

This is well described with minocycline and with other drugs including chlorpromazine, isoniazid, procainamide, penicillamine, hydralazine and methyl-dopa.

Drug-induced lupus occurs in individuals with a genetic predisposition. The clinical and immunological features are similar to those of idiopathic SLE. Classically, the double stranded DNA binding is negative and anti-histone antibodies are often detectable unlike idiopathic lupus where only 25 per cent have detectable levels. Minocycline induced SLE may be serologically similar to idiopathic lupus. The sex ratio is equal compared with the 13:1 female to male ratio in idiopathic disease.

Treatment:

The principle of management is to withdraw the offending drug and to take care when prescribing other implicated drugs in the future. Steroids may be necessary to treat the clinical manifestations. The immunological abnormalities will resolve spontaneously.

CASE 20

The following photograph and series of radiographs belong to a 62-year-old man with longstanding back pain.

Describe the characteristic features shown in the photograph.

Describe the radiological abnormalities.

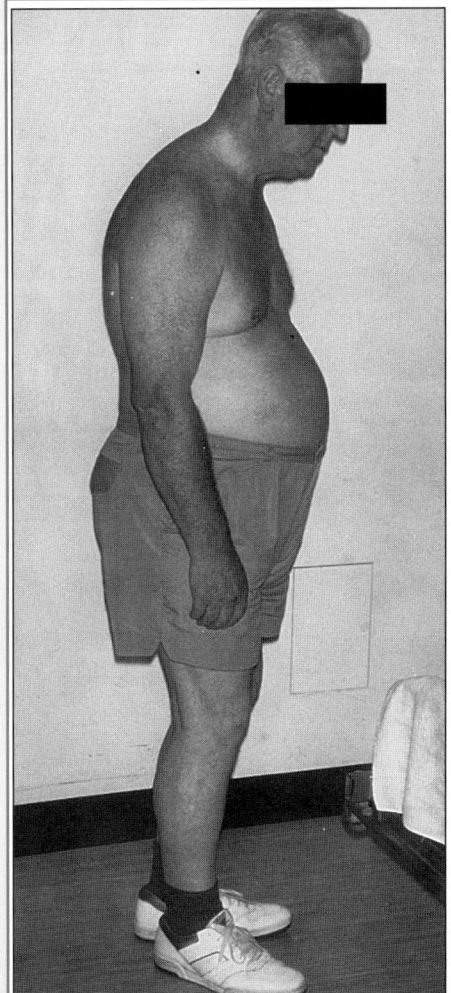

Middle-aged man with ankylosing spondylitis

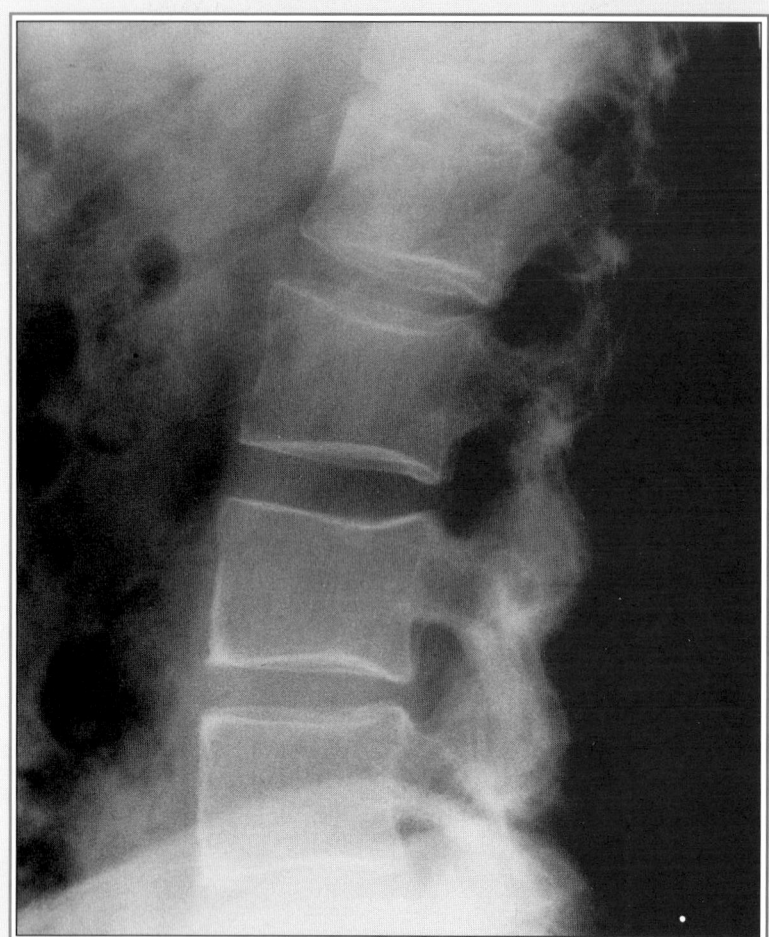

Figure 1

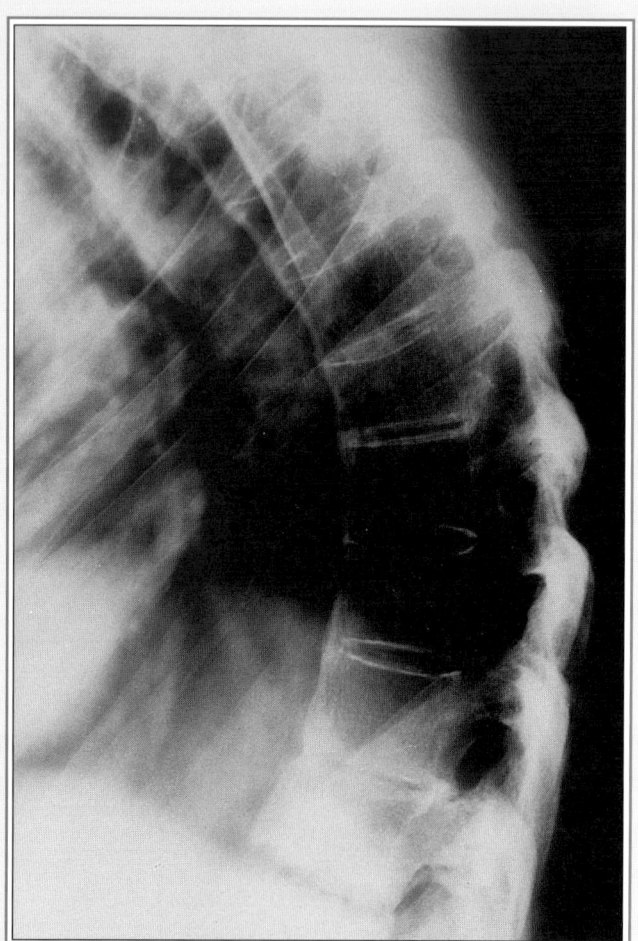

Figure 2: (at a later stage in his disease)

66

Answer to Case 20

Figure 1, shows the squaring of the lower lumbar vertebrae with Romanus lesion of the anterosuperior and anteinferior margins leading to the loss of the normal concavity of the anterior aspect of the vertebral body. Figure 2, shows the bamboo spine produced by bridging ossification of the invertebral ligaments.

The patient demonstrates a loss of lumbar lordosis, increased thoracic kyphosis and a compensatory increase in cervical extension. His abdomen is protuberant because of the increased diaphragmatic respiration needed to oxygenate his lungs in the face of a mechanical failure of chest expansion. On examination, the patient had a loss of spinal movement in all directions suggesting an inflammatory process as opposed to a mechanical one (loss of lateral flexion is a very early and characteristic sign). The diagnosis is ankylosing spondylitis.

The radiographic features of the condition are as follows:

- Sacroiliitis - loss of the joint space with irregularity, erosions and sclerosis, and finally ankylosis leading to fusion
- Squaring of the vertebrae
- Romanus lesions (inflammatory lesions that are seen as an erosive defect on the anterior border of the vertebra adjacent to the disc)
- Apophyseal joint ankylosis (fusion of facet joints)
- Calcification of the paraspinal ligaments
- Formation of syndesmophytes (calcification of the outer surfaces of the discs).

Ultimately, calcification of the paraspinal ligaments, fusion of the facet joints and the bony bridging between vertebrae produces a rigid ankylosed spine. The radiological appearances are often described as a bamboo or poker spine.

The following complications may occur:

1) Directly related to spinal disease -
- Spinal fracture
- Radiculopathy
- Mechanical failure of ventilation.
2) Other joint involvement -
- Peripheral large joint arthropathy usually shoulders, hips and knees.
3) Extra articular manifestations of the disease -
- Anterior uveitis
- Pulmonary upper lobe fibrosis
- Aortitis.

Therapy of established ankylosing spondylitis aims to maintain mobility and functional capacity as described in Case 3. This is achieved by physiotherapy used in conjunction with NSAIDs to suppress pain and inflammation. Disease modifying drugs, such as sulphasalazine or methotrexate are useful in suppressing inflammation, particularly in affected peripheral joints.

Anterior uveitis may be treated using topical steroid drops.

CASE 21

Tanya, a 32-year-old hairdresser, had a two day history of pain and swelling of both ankles. She developed the rash shown this morning and visited your clinic.

Which investigations would you request?

What is the diagnosis?

What treatment is appropriate?

What other skin manifestations can this condition have?

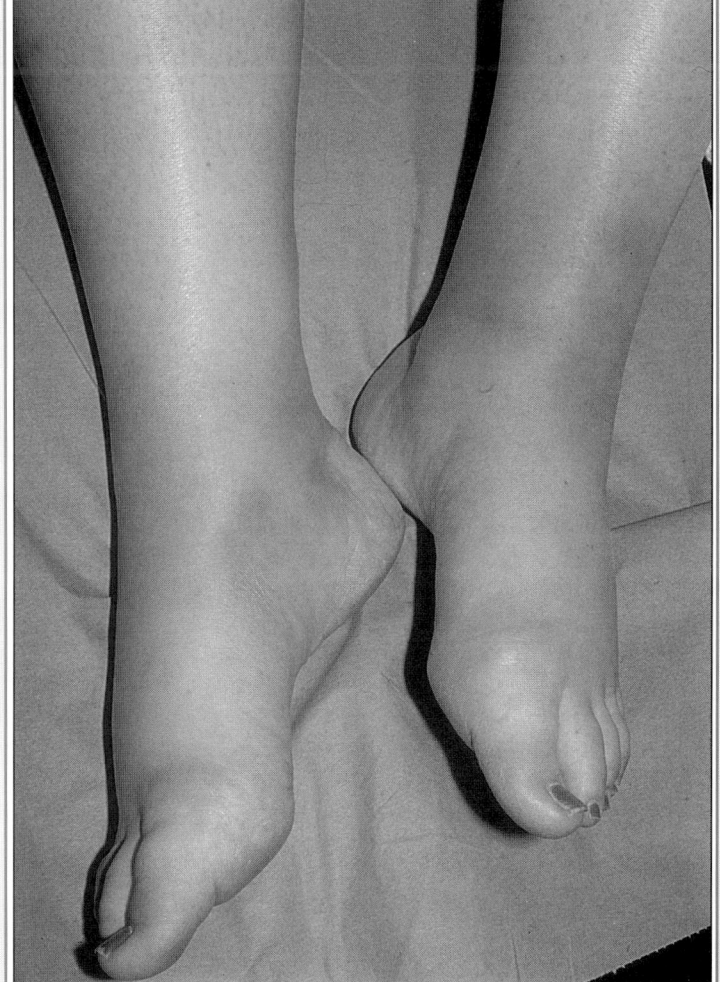

Figure 1

Answer to Case 21

The chest X-ray shows bilateral hila lymphadenopathy. She has erythema nodosum on her shins. The most likely diagnosis is sarcoidosis.

This condition should be suspected in any young adult presenting with acute polyarthritis in the presence of erythema nodosum. Monoarthritis is very unusual. The joints most frequently affected by this non-destructive synovitis are knees, ankles, wrists, elbows and proximal interphalangeal joints. A chest X-ray will confirm the presence of bilateral hila lymphadenopathy in about 90 per cent of cases. This is associated with a good prognosis but the outlook is worse if there are pulmonary infiltrates, fibrosis or bullae formation. The arthritis will resolve within four months but resolution can be hastened by treatment with oral or intra-articular corticosteroids.

Investigations will show elevation of the ESR and CRP and 15 per cent of sufferers can be rheumatoid factor positive. The serum angiotensin converting enzyme level (ACE) may be elevated because of increased ACE production from within the non-caseating granulomas which characterise the histological appearance of sarcoidosis. Hypercalcuria due to vitamin D sensitivity is common, although hypercalcaemia is rare except when dehydrated. The cause of sarcoidosis is not known. The classical skin manifestation of chronic sarcoidosis is *lupus pernio*.

The investigations should be:
Chest X-ray.
Serum angiotensin converting enzyme level serum calcium.

Your diagnosis should be:
Acute Sarcoidosis (erythema nodosum, synovitis, bilateral hila lymphadenopathy constitutes Lofgren's Syndrome).

Treatment should be:
Oral corticosteroids together with simple analgesics or non-steroidal anti-inflammatory agents.

Other skin manifestations:
Lupus pernio.

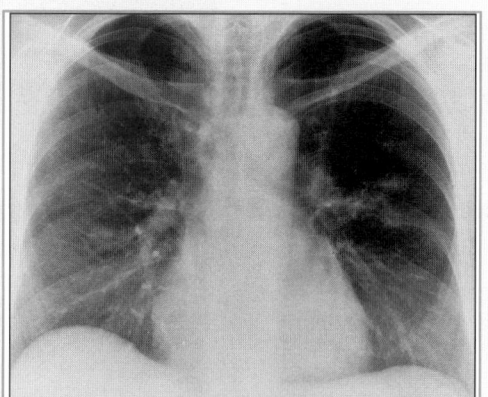

Chest X-ray

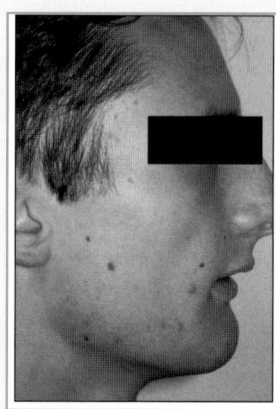

Lupus pernio

CASE 22

Marjorie is 55 years old and was diagnosed as having rheumatoid arthritis four years ago. She has been treated with NSAIDs but recently has become increasingly symptomatic with stiffness lasting all day. Indeed, she had to be carried off the aircraft on her return home from a trip abroad.

A week ago, she noticed that her right foot was beginning to drag when she walked and she began to experience numbness and tingling in her right hand. Initially, these symptoms were attributed to a stroke and she was admitted to hospital for investigations.

On examination, Majorie had a widespread active symmetrical synovitis with nodules on both elbows. Her right index finger had been cold and discoloured for 24 hours. Neurological examination revealed altered sensation in all fingers of her right hand and an inability to dorsiflex her right ankle.

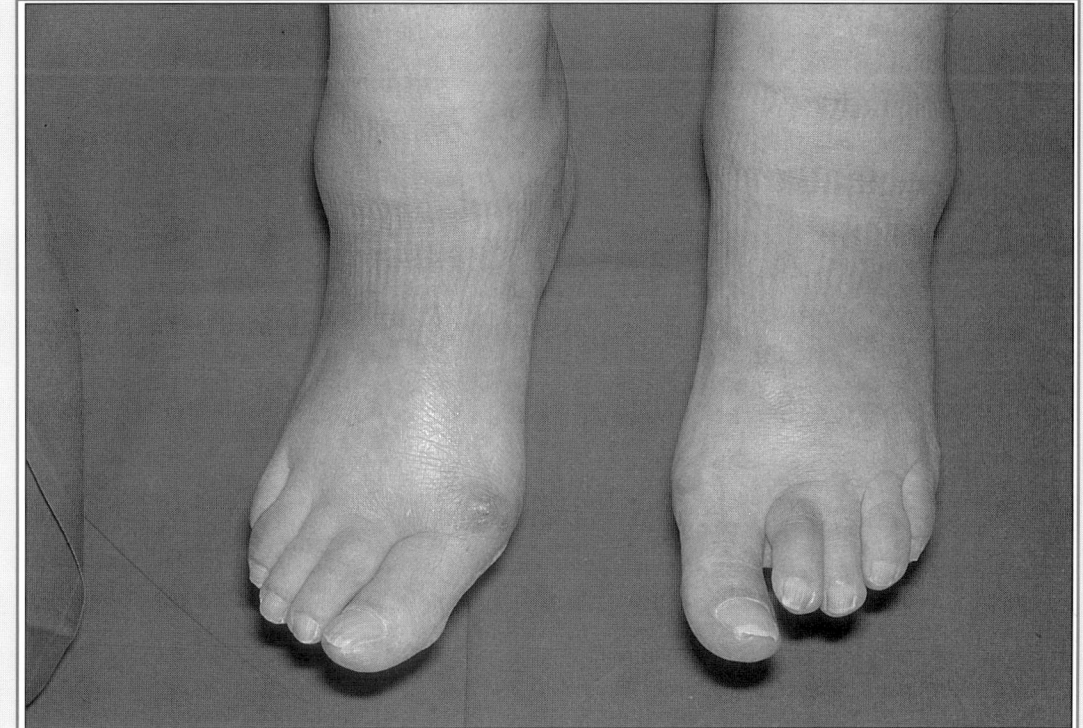

Figure 1

What is the most likely cause of neurological abnormalities in her hands and feet.

What is the significance of her ischaemic finger?

What is the underlying diagnosis?

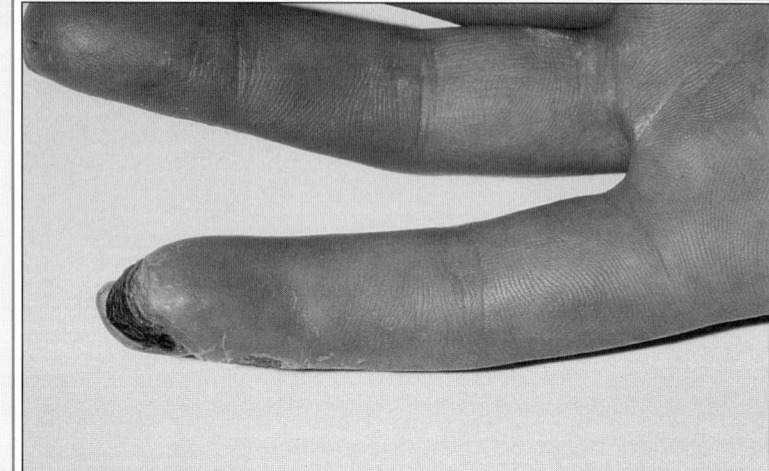

Figure 2

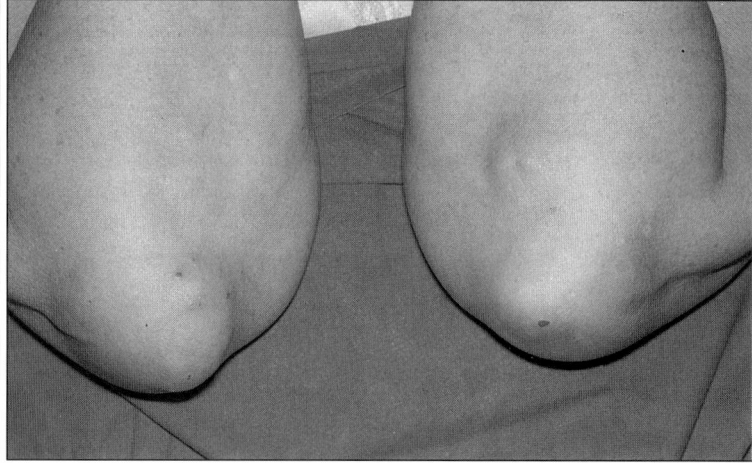

Figure 3

Answer to Case 22

Marjorie has footdrop due to a lesion in the lateral popliteal nerve. This can be distinguished from an S1 root lesion (which would also produce footdrop), because the only area supplied by the lateral popliteal nerve is between the first and second toes, whereas the dermatomal distribution of S1 is across the plantar surface of the foot extending proximally a short way up the flexor aspect of the leg.

The neurological symptoms in her right hand were due to carpal tunnel syndrome.

Figure 1 shows bilateral ankle joint swelling due to synovitis. Figure 2 shows evidence of finger pulp infarction. Figure 3 shows a number of vasculitic lesions over the elbows and a right olecranon bursitis.

A unifying diagnosis to explain all of these abnormalities is that she has developed rheumatoid vasculitis. Vasculitis of the blood supply to the peripheral nerves (vasa nervorum) and digital arteries has resulted in the development of mononeuritis multiplex and finger pulp infarction respectively.

Vasculitis is a complication of established RA and is particularly associated with a high titre rheumatoid factor.

The patient should be immunosuppressed; one possibility is IV therapy with a combination of methylprednisolone and cyclophosphamide.

Nerve condition studies can be used to locate the sites of nerve involvement. These can be treated with local infiltration of hydrocortisone around the nerve. Appliances such as subtalar supports and physiotherapy can help to improve the gait.

CASE 23

What abnormalities can you see in this X-ray of the cervical spine?

What is the investigation of choice?

What neurological signs would you expect to find in the upper limbs on examination?

This patient has chronic rheumatoid arthritis. The staff nurse telephones to tell you that the patient has become incontinent of urine. What will you do?

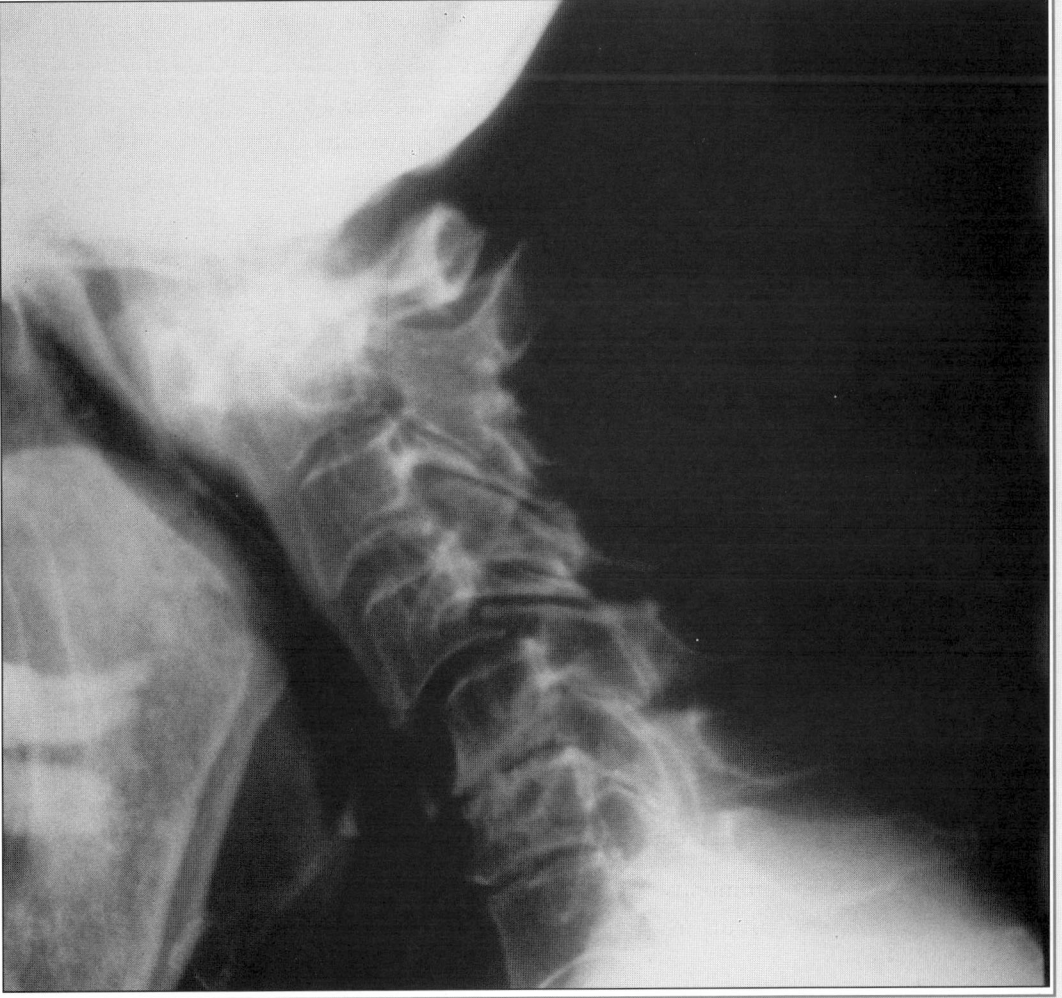

X-ray: cervical spine

Answer to Case 23

The X-ray shows evidence of atlanto-axial instability and an anterior slip of C4 on C5. Atlantoaxial instability is primarily due to instability of the transverse ligaments which hold the odontoid peg to the atlas.

The symptoms described in this case are of cervical cord compression due to vertebral instability.

1. Evidence of bilateral upper motor neurone signs with increased tone (often with sustained clonus), decreased muscle power, brisk reflexes and extensor plantar responses.

2. Evidence of a sensory level.

3. Loss of bladder and bowel control.

Atlantoaxial instability is due to erosion of the transverse ligament of the atlas. This ligament holds the odontoid peg against the anterior inner surface of the atlas. If the ligament is damaged, during cervical flexion, the odontoid pig is able to move posteriorly and may compress the cord against the posterior surface of the atlas. This can be seen on a cervical spine X-ray, with the neck in flexion, when the space between the anterior surface of the odontoid peg and the anterior inner surface of the atlas is more than 3mm (see diagram opposite).

This situation is an emergency as without treatment to relieve the cord compression, irreversible paraplegia may develop. A neurosurgical procedure may be required to stabilise the vertebra and prevent further compression of the spinal cord.

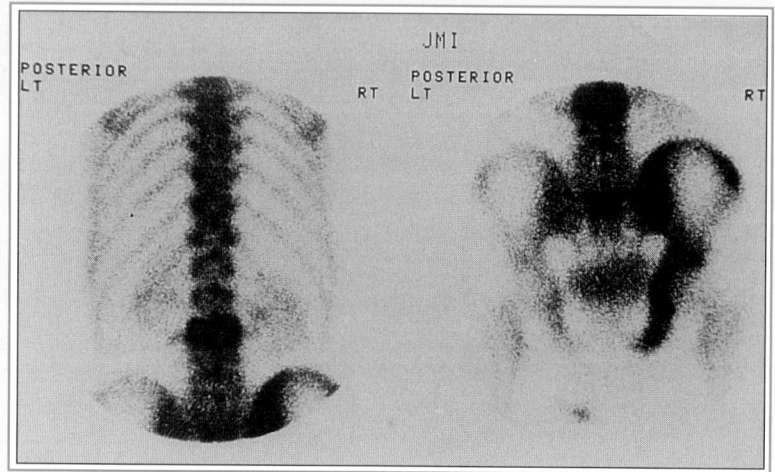

CASE 24

An elderly lady presents to emergency having collapsed at home. She gives a three day history of increasingly severe pain in her left wrist. She had been unable to use the hand for 24 hours. There is no history of injury to her wrist.

On admission, she was pyrexial with a temperature of 39°C. She had features of generalised osteoarthritis and a hot swollen left wrist.

What is the diagnosis?

What investigations should be performed?

What is the treatment?

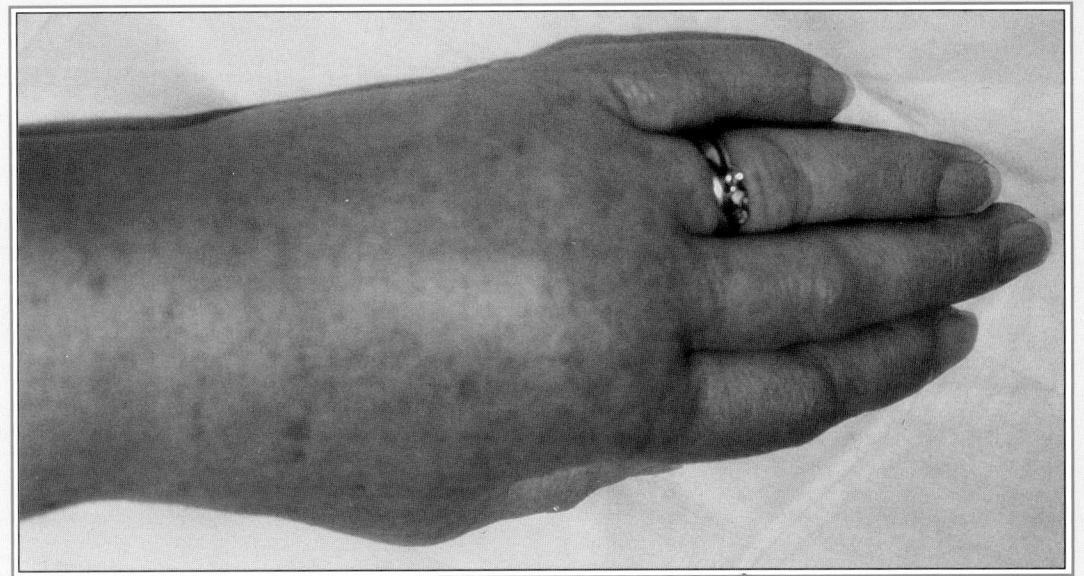

Answer to Case 24

The most likely diagnosis is septic arthritis of the left wrist. Other possible diagnoses include gout and pseudogout. A fracture should be excluded by the X-ray.

The following investigations/procedures should be performed:

◆ Full blood count and urea and electrolytes

◆ Blood cultures

◆ X-ray of joint

◆ Aspirate joint and culture the fluid obtained

◆ ± Synovial biopsy.

A negative synovial fluid culture does not exclude infection, especially for acid fast bacilli and where this diagnosis is suspected, a biopsy should be considered.

Septic arthritis requires treatment with intravenous antibiotics combined with joint drainage. The choice of antibiotic is dependent on the organism concerned. The most common infecting organism is staphylococcus aureus which is often treated using a combination of high dose intravenous flucloxacillin and oral fusidic acid. The flucloxacillin should be given intravenously in order to effectively penetrate the synovial membrane.

A septic joint requires daily aspiration and lavage if possible. With a wrist joint this is most easily achieved by needle aspiration. However if a large joint is involved, for example the hip, surgical drainage is required.

CASE 25

Jim, a 62-year-old company director, has been under your care for the last three years with hypertension for which he receives a thiazide diuretic.

He presents with sudden onset of severe pain in his foot. On direct questioning, he comments that he is becoming increasingly tired, feels mentally slower than he used to be and is struggling to cope with his work. He complains that he always feels cold.

What are the diagnoses?

What investigations are indicated?

What is the treatment?

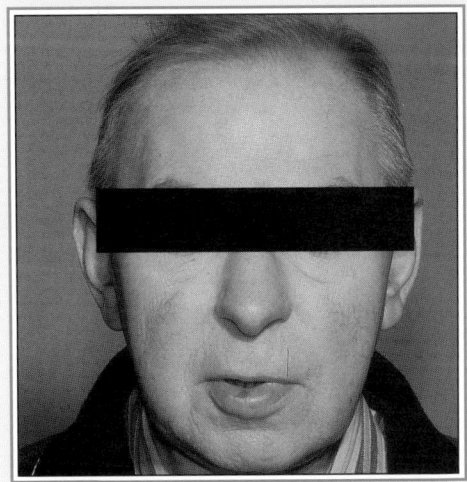

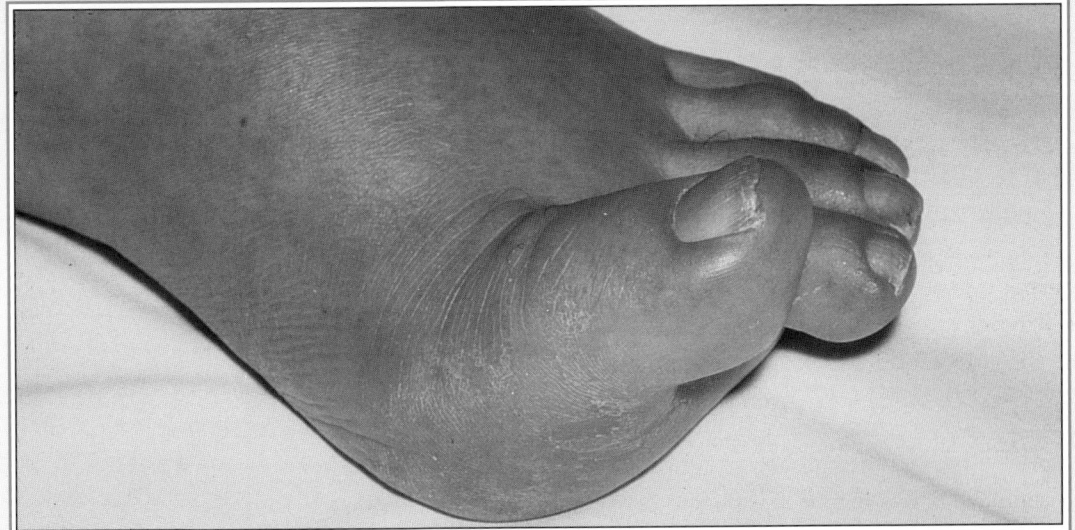

Answer to Case 25

Gout is responsible for the pain in the foot. The pain and inflammation of gout is caused by the deposition of crystals of monosodium urate within the joint and surrounding soft tissues. There are two stages in the natural history of the disease. Initially, the patient suffers with recurrent attacks of arthritis with full resolution. However, in the later stages the attacks fail to resolve completely and there are persistent symptoms associated with permanent deposition of urate in the joint.

A number of conditions predispose to the development of gout; these are shown in the Table. In this case, Jim is hypothyroid and on a thiazide diuretic, both of which predispose to the development of gout.

The following investigations should be performed:

♦ Serum urate

♦ Thyroid function tests

♦ X-ray of ankle

♦ Aspiration of ankle joint and fluid sent for microscopy and culture and crystals.

Acute attack

Acute attacks are treated with NSAIDs, for example indomethacin 50 mg tds or piroxicam 40 mg o.d. If patients are intolerant of NSAIDs, oral colchicine can be used on a short term basis. It is effective but causes diarrhoea with high doses. In addition, the joint can be injected with a steroid preparation.

Long term therapy

Risk factors for the condition should be identified. In this case the hypothyroidism should be treated and the thiazide diuretic withdrawn.

Allopurinol is the drug of choice to prevent recurrent attacks. This is an inhibitor of the enzyme xanthine oxidase which is responsible for the production of urate. Allopurinol should not be started within four weeks of an attack because it may precipitate a further one. If it has to be commenced urgently it should be combined with a NSAID. Azapropazone may have a special role as a uricosuric NSAID.

CAUSES OF HYPERURICAEMIA	
Impaired excretion of uric acid	**Overproduction of uric acid**
Idiopathic	Idiopathic
Thiazide diuretic	Increased purine turnover
Low dose aspirin	Myeloproliferative disorder
Hypothyroidism	Lymphoproliferative disorder
Primary hyperparathyroidism	Severe psoriasis
Alcohol	
Lead toxicity	
Chronic renal disease	

Purines are constituents of the DNA backbone. They are broken down to be excreted as urates.

CASE 26

Dave, a 52-year-old man, presents with a two month history of increasing weakness of his shoulder and hips associated with increasing tiredness. His past medical history is unremarkable. He is a smoker but does not have any respiratory symptoms, apart from a morning cough.

On examination, he has a rash around his eyes and at the back of his hands. In addition, there is marked weakness of his shoulder and pelvic girdle.

What diagnosis do you suspect?

What investigations do you perform?

What is the treatment?

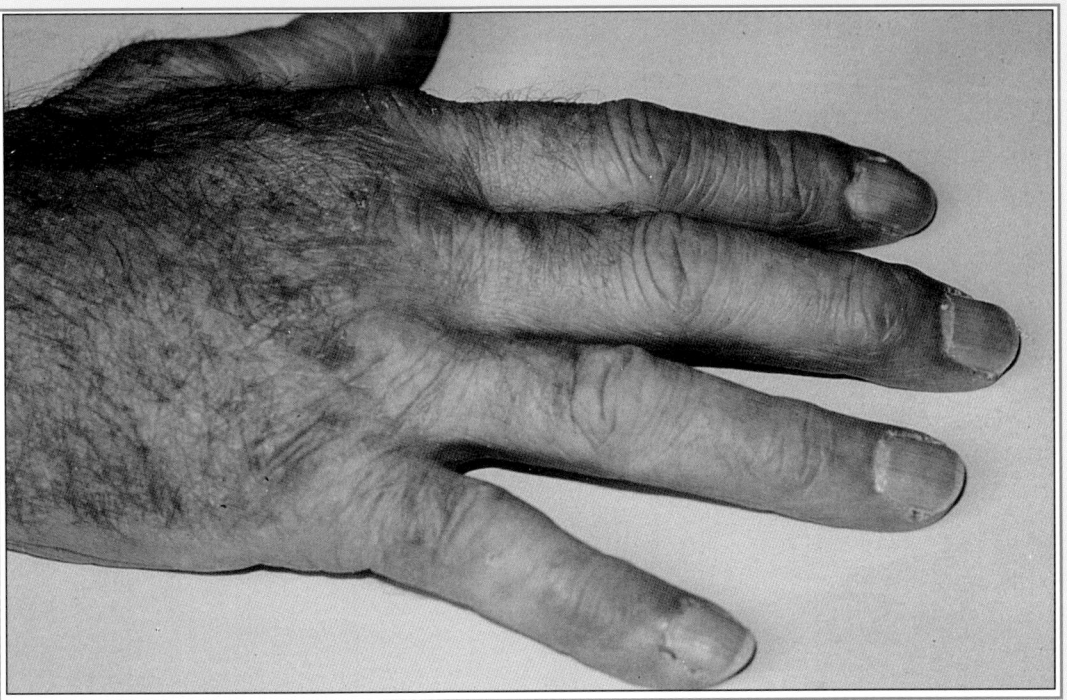

Answer to Case 26

The most likely diagnosis is dermatomyositis. The patient has the characteristic rash of the condition on his face and hands. The rash is described as 'heliotrop' on the face and the nodules on the hands are called 'Gottrons papules', as shown overleaf.

In adults, this condition can occur as a non metastatic manifestation of malignancy and this must be borne in mind (the childhood condition is not associated with malignancy). The most commonly associated malignancies are carcinoma of the bronchus, breast, large bowel, prostate and ovary.

The following investigations are required to make the diagnosis:

◆ Muscle enzymes - raised and CK and AST proportional to disease activity

◆ Electromyograph - consistent with acute myositis

◆ Autoantibody screen - Rhf 50% ANA 30% including anti Jo-1 antibody

◆ Renal profile

◆ Muscle BX - evidence of muscle fibre degeneration/ regeneration and fibrosis.

In addition, these tests are required to exclude internal malignancy:

◆ Chest X-ray

◆ Ultrasound

◆ Ultrascan of abdomen and pelvis

◆ Mammography

◆ Barium enema

◆ Prostate specific antigen and ultrasound of prostate.

In the case presented, a chest X-ray showed a clinically unsuspected carcinoma of the bronchus.

Treatment is clearly dependent on whether the condition is associated with malignant disease or not. If it is present, it will require treatment which may result in improvement in the dermatomyositis. In those conditions not associated with malignant disease, the mainstay of treatment is oral prednisolone, usually combined with azathioprine or methotrexate.

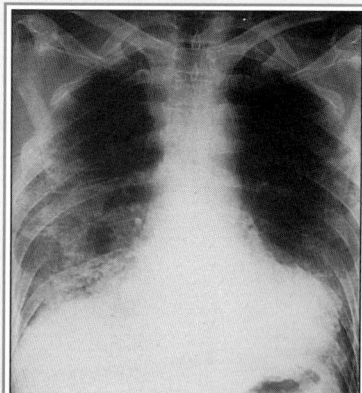

Chest X-ray showing right lower zone shadowing which turned out to be due to a proximal cancer of the bronchus causing a pneumonia distally

A 27-year-old Mediterranean university student presents to emergency with blurring of vision, bilateral knee pain and swelling, and painful bruising on his legs.

12 months ago he had been admitted with 'meningitis' and deep venous thrombosis of the left leg. He has had recurrent mouth and scrotal ulcers since the age 21.

On examination, he has bilateral hypopyo uveitis, bilateral knee arthritis, erythema nodosum over the shins and a few mouth ulcers. Investigations: Hb 12.5 g/dl; plasma viscosity 1.82; Rheumatoid factor -ve; ANF -ve; Chest radiograph - normal.

What is the most likely diagnosis?

What additional test might confirm the diagnosis?

What is the most frequent, serious manifestation?

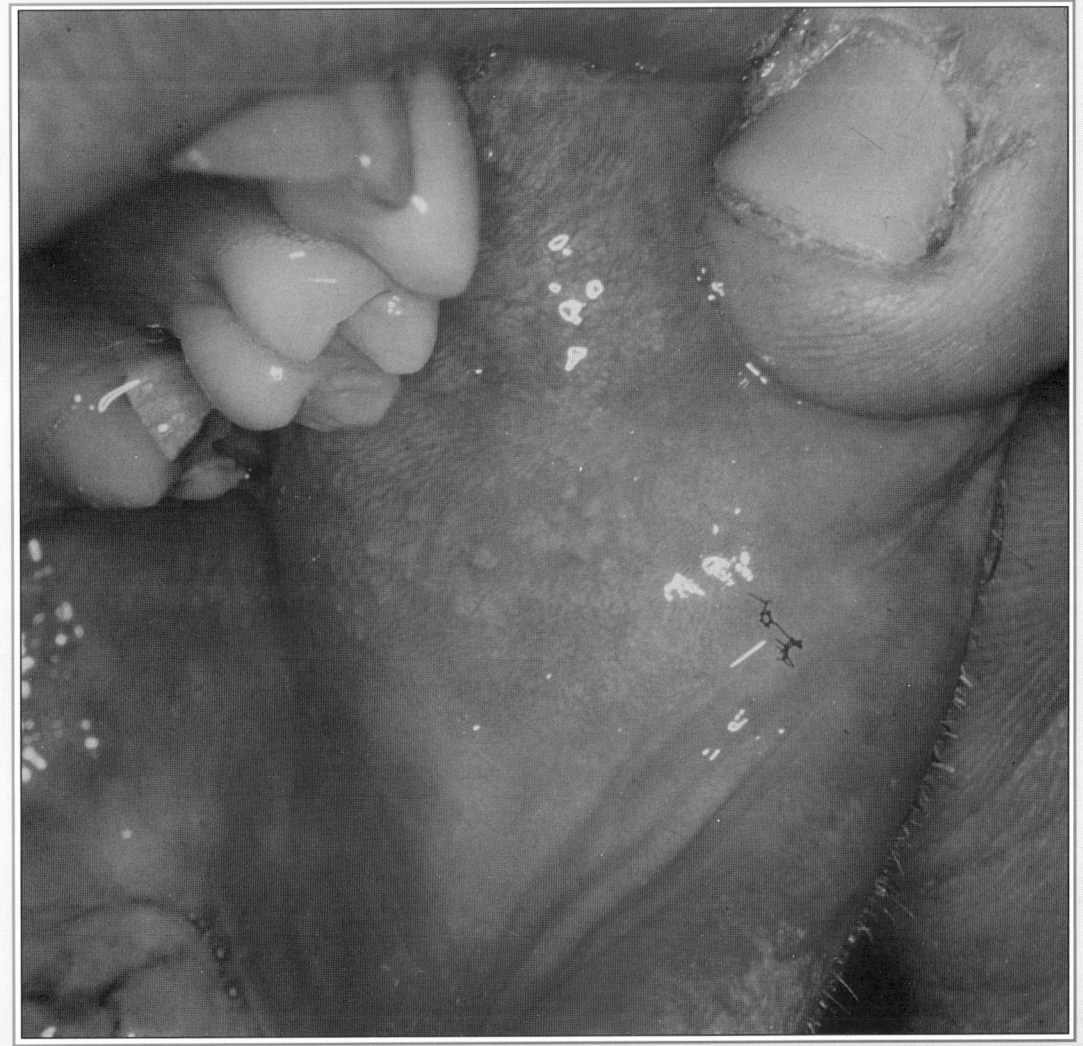

Answer to Case 27

Behcet's Disease is a multisystem vasculitic disorder characterised by recurrent oral and genital ulceration, uveitis, acneiform or papopustular skin lesions. Erythema nodosum and non-erosive arthritis are other common features. Peripheral and central venous and arterial occlusion, small and large intestine inflammation, stroke and meningoencephalitis are rarer manifestations.

The pathology is of systemic vasculitis with venous thrombosis formation. Some patients have skin hyperreactivity to minor trauma such as at needle venepuncture sites. This is the basis for the pathergy reaction which occurs almost exclusively in Behcet's Disease. This phenomenon is, however, uncommon in patients with Behcet's Disease in Northern Europe and America.

The clinical criteria for diagnosis are the presence of recurrent oral ulcers and two of the following: recurrent genital ulceration, uveitis, typical skin lesions (acneiform lesions not erythema nodosum), the presence of the pathergy reaction. The mean age of onset is between 25 and 35. The male to female ratio is approximately 1:1, although men tend to develop more severe disease. Behcet's Disease occurs mainly in the Mediterranean countries (Turkey, Middle East and the Far East (China, Japan), where it is associated with HLA B51. It occurs rarely in Northern Europe and America. The prevalence rate varies from 10/100,000 in Japan to 300/100,000 in Turkey.

The most frequent serious manifestation of Behcet's Disease is eye involvement which occurs in up to 60 per cent of patients. It can lead to blindness and requires urgent immunosuppressive treatment. Prednisolone, azathioprine and cyclosporin are the mainstays for treatment. Colchicine is used for mouth and genital ulceration, and joint manifestations. Large vessel thrombosis requires anticoagulation and immunosuppression.

An additional test which might help confirm Behcet's Disease is a pathergy test.

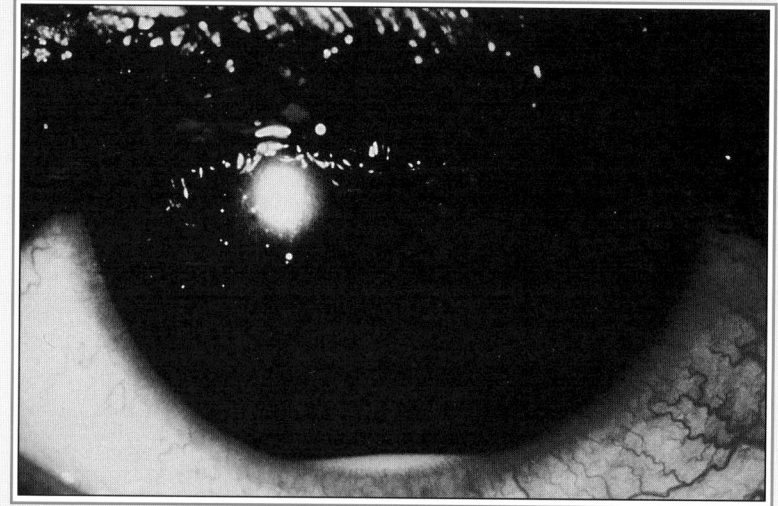

Hyphaema in Behcet's Disease

Abbreviations used in the text:

ANA	Antinuclear antibody
ANCA	Antineutrophil cytoplasmic antibody
AST	Aspartate transaminase
AVN	Antivascular necrosis
CK	Creatine phosphokinase
CRP	C-reactive protein
CT Scan	Computerised tomographic scan
dsDNA	Double stranded DNA antibody
ESR	Erythrocyte sedimentation rate
RA	Rheumatoid arthritis
SIJ	Sacroiliac joints
SLE	Systemic lupus erythematosus
US	Ultrasound

Further reading:

Oxford Textbook of Rheumatology
Oxford Medical Publications 1993
PJ Maddison, DA Isenberg, P Woo, DN Glass.

Lecture Notes in Rheumatology
Blackwell Scientific Publications 1985
J Edmonds, G Hughes.

Connective Tissue Diseases
Blackwell Scientific Publications 1994
G. Hughes.

Medicine (Rheumatology Volumes)
The Medicine Group.

Illustrated Case Histories in Rheumatology
Mosby-Wolfe 1995
L. Hordon, A. Isdale, H. Bird.

Essentials of Rheumatology
Churchill Livingstone 1988
H. Currey.